Live Life in Full Color

A practical guide to balancing your chakras for optimal well-being

Catherine Shovlin

Context

This book is dedicated to

every colorful, life affirming character

I have met along the way

By the same author

Your True Colors

*A practical guide to applying color psychology in your
life*

Walking through Walls

Proactively challenging barriers in ourselves and society

Live Life in Full Color
An introduction to working with your chakras

By Catherine Shovlin

Table of Contents

WHY: ...   **6**

PART 1: ...   **10**

Context   11

Our anatomy – physical and subtle   12

What are chakras exactly?   15

Healing our chakras   20

HOW: ...   **23**

How to work with your chakras   24

Chakra meditation   25

Root chakra   32

Sacral chakra   46

Solar plexus chakra   64

Context

Heart chakra · 80

Throat chakra · 105

Third eye chakra · 125

Crown chakra · 144

INTEGRATION... · 167

Your chakra journey · 168

CLOSING WORDS... · 185

Your journey from here · 185

Gratitudes · 187

INDEX : · 189

Why: ...

Foreword: My own story

Why: ...Context

More than 6 billion people on the planet. How many of them are full of life? I'm not talking about how many are sick or compromised in some way, but how many just go from day to day, following their routines. Saying things like "how can it be New Year already! It seems five minutes since the last one?" Responding to an enquiry as to how they are with an automatic and empty "Fine".

Maybe you feel like that sometimes. Trudging through the chores, waiting for the train, waiting for Friday, waiting for pay day, waiting for the holidays.

I have certainly been like that at times. In survival mode. Forgetting really that I am actually alive in this moment, and that life is a gift. I consider myself fortunate though that on my journey through life I have come across some teachings and some teachers that have opened my eyes. And my mind and my heart!

An important key for me has been getting to know my chakras – working with them so they can work with me. They have helped me feel more clear-headed, more energized, more open-hearted and just more alive.

In this book I will share with you some of the information that I have found useful about what chakras are, how they work and what you can do to enhance their contribution to your physical and emotional well-being.

But first I want to share with you how I got to know them in the first place, and how they have helped me.

Let's roll back three decades.

I felt a distinct buzzing under my finger as I passed over Angela's eyebrow. That sensation made no sense to my mathematician's logical, analytical mind but I could feel it so I made small circles as instructed to see if I could stop it.

Suddenly Angela gasped and doubled up in pain. We looked at each other in alarm. What had I done?

It turned out that Angela had gall stones and the buzzing I felt under her skin was at her gall bladder point (according to reflexology systems).

I was, frankly, amazed. My head was spinning with the implications. It seemed to suggest firstly that this idea of points on your face (or hands or feet) really did represent parts of your body – I had considered it all rather fanciful till then. And – more alarmingly – it suggested that I could somehow sense that. And affect it.

Seeing the looks on both our faces, Sarah, our teacher, reassured us that I hadn't done any harm, just unblocked some energy which had caused the release of pain and probably a shift in the state of the gallstones (for the better). My partner confirmed that in fact now she was over the initial shock, she felt better than she had for weeks.

That one incident changed my view completely. Over my journey of the next thirty years, from the more tangible holistic massage training I did soon after, through reflexology, reiki, yoga, sound healing, aura reading and shamanic healing practices, I have developed a strong and deepening respect for the energy channels in our bodies.

I now see my physical body more like the flame of a candle. It has a definite visible core – the part we refer to as our body because we can see it and touch it – but it also has a much wider effect, a zone of influence.

The warmth and the light that it generates spread much further. Helping to explain how some people seem "larger than life" while others look diminished and shrink into themselves.

One of the most accessible aspects of this bigger self is our chakras. They anchor the energetic body to the physical one. They manifest in our physical bodies and they give us a way to quickly shift how energy is moving – or not moving – around us.

They have so many gifts for us if we just take a little care of them – they are still surprising me! And I am excited to share some of this with you, explaining a little of the technicalities and also offering ways to tune up your chakras and unleash more of your own magnificence.

Now let's get started on turning up the color in your life, increasing your vitality and sense of well-being for your sake and the sake of everybody around you.

With very best wishes

Catherine, Ubud, Bali, May 2020

Part 1: …

What are chakras and why do they matter?

Context

Many ancient traditions around the world refer to our energetic body. This is something that is part of us in the same way as our physical body. In fact, you might say the physical body is that part of the body that is in the range of the electromagnetic spectrum that is visible to us.

As we know, the rainbow that we can see doesn't stop where we can no longer see it. But rather continues to infra-red and beyond at one end and ultraviolet and beyond at the other.

Likewise, our holistic body also includes invisible aspects.

This doesn't take a leap of faith to contemplate. A simple example is the heat emanating from your body. We can all feel and accept that aspect of energy around our physical form even though we can't see it unless we have access to an infrared camera.

I was surprised to learn that as long as 100 years ago the medical profession were developing scientific instruments to measure the energy field around every human.

They discovered that this was measurable and that there was a specific wavelength frequency or range of frequencies (Hertz, like we know from tuning the radio) for each different organ. In the same way as we measure the frequency of other parts of the electromagnetic spectrum such as musical notes within the sound wave section, colors within the visible light section, x-rays, microwaves, gamma rays and so on, they could identify the frequency emitted by our organs.

And then of course there is our emotional understanding of our energetic body. When we speak of magnetic attraction, or someone giving off a bad vibe – or a good one - we are referring, maybe unconsciously, to our awareness of this other level of our existence.

Our anatomy – physical and subtle

Concept

Let us consider then that as well as our physical body we also have an energetic one. As with our physical body, this subtle or energetic body has some structures and systems, and can be in a healthy state, or struggling.

The primary energetic structure is that of meridians – the equivalent of our heart, arteries and veins for blood, the nerves and nervous system for information or the lymph system for cleansing waste products and toxins from our body.

Medical practices such as acupuncture, acupressure, and reflexology draw most obviously on this, though all healing practices have some relationship with our energetic body, including the placebo effect referred to by pharmaceutical medicine.

Although this may have been dismissed as an amusing observation of human nature in the past, it is now beginning to be respected as an aspect of healing.

As well as the measured placebo effect, there is also a nocebo component whereby somebody given the same drugs for their condition, but told they have just received a placebo, does not manifest the same response as those who knowingly receive the same drug.

Let's take a look at the structure of this alternative information system running through our bodies. And see how it relates to the chakras.

Meridians

The diagram shows the central meridian system and how the chakras attach to it.

- The central meridian, the *sushumna nadi*, runs from the tailbone to the top of the head and has four meridians running alongside it (those behind the sushumna and to the right of it for masculine or yang energy, those in front and to the left for feminine or yin energy).
- We also have peripheral meridians relating to our organs and bodily functions eg lung meridian, colon meridian. Each has their own particular route through the body. If you have ever experienced reflexology then your therapist would have been working via these meridians.
- The chakras are those points on the body where these meridians or energetic pathways interact with our physical systems. They are also considered to be access points for external energetic systems and healing to take place, for example using reiki or yoga.

What are chakras exactly?

The role of chakras

We can think of chakras as intersections or junctions. Places where information and energy can be exchanged and communicated between our physical anatomy and our energetic or subtle anatomy (you might sometimes also hear it being called esoteric). Also, where either of these bodies can communicate with the outside world.

If you imagine this as a road system, and each chakra as a roundabout / traffic circle / rotary, then it is easy to see why we would want them to be as clean and clear as possible. Anybody who has to drive a route with a number of these type of junctions will know only too well how frustrating they can be when they get backed up with traffic and everyone is blocking everyone else.

In many practices such as yoga, meditation and the martial arts, based on Eastern philosophy, good chakra maintenance is a prerequisite for a healthy and powerful body as well as a good mental state and access to other aspects of our humanity such as creativity, compassion and the spiritual realm.

As you see in the diagram they are often portrayed as cones or vortices. Drawing in energy and spinning to give it the impetus it needs to move up and down the central meridian. Many practices aim to stimulate and/or balance this energetic flow to improve our overall well-being.

Where can I find my chakras?

Referring again to our diagram, you see that this book is based on the seven-chakra system. You may come across versions with fewer, or more chakras, but I will focus on seven - the most widely used system and one you might hear mentioned for example in your yoga class.

In general, we start at the bottom, the root chakra, and work our way up to the top one - the crown chakra. It is easiest to consider them as situated in the center of your physical body. So, although we might for example place a hand on our chest to indicate the heart chakra, it is equally accessible from the back of our body, between the shoulder blades.

It is helpful to be familiar with the locations of your chakras if you aren't already. If you want to work with them, it gives you a focus for your attention to know their location. You can get a general idea from the earlier diagram, and in Part 2 of this book where we look at the chakras one by one, you will find a lot more information about each chakra, including their location.

What do chakras do?

As mentioned already, you can think of chakras as junctions on the energetic superhighway known in Sanskrit as *sushumna nadi*.

The better they flow, they better the energy flows. When they are congested or even blocked then that has consequences for our state of mind as well as our physical health and general attitude to life.

We all have to deal with some knockbacks in our lives – from trivial issues like the coffee machine playing up, to major trauma or bereavement.

Sometimes these events are personal to you and those near to you, other times they may be society-wide for example a war, a natural disaster or a pandemic. In these systemic cases not only can we use our chakra awareness to take care of ourselves but also to make a positive contribution to the overall energetic field of our whole community or society.

Good chakra health may not change *the events* that happen in our lives, but in can help us in how we *respond* to the challenges that life throws at us.

Well balanced chakras can help us be more like *okiagari*, the Japanese dolls with such a low center of gravity they cannot be knocked over. The *Weeble* toys popular in the west follow the same principle. "Weebles wobble but they don't fall down." This kind of resilience and equanimity is invaluable in coping with the ups and downs of life with grace.

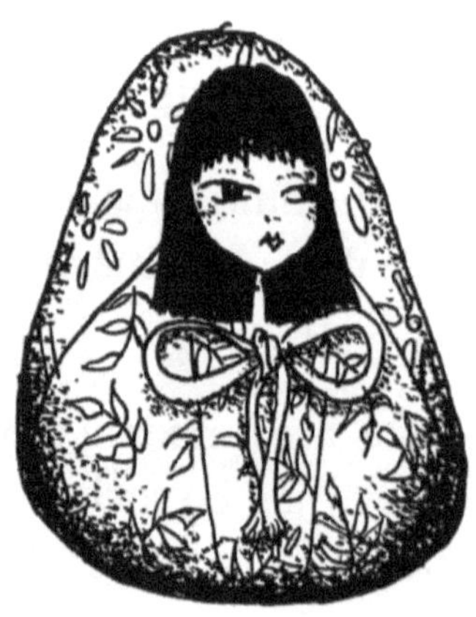

Yoga guidance

You will see that I have included a few yoga postures in each chakra chapter. These instructions may be enough for you.

If you would like a bit more visual guidance, then you can find this in three places:

- my website windsofdiscovery.com/chakras
- my YouTube channel (youtube.com/CatherineShovlin)
- the Winds of Discovery app, available in the Apple and Google stores

You will find a short video there for each chakra - with the yoga moves described in this book – as well as the guided meditations.

You may also enjoy some of the additional material available on my YouTube channel like the 21 Day "FreeTreat" series with suggestions, guided meditations and breathing exercises to increase equanimity and resilience in times of trouble. These videos were developed during the COVID-19 pandemic but would apply equally to any other especially challenging time in your life.

A note of caution

Please be mindful that the practices in this book may release long held (and no longer valid for you) limiting beliefs, fears and emotions.

Take care of yourself on this chakra journey and get the support you need as and when things arise. There's no rush. You've had your chakras all your life, so you don't need to 'fix' them in two days. Go at your own pace and enjoy the journey.

Know also that this is an ongoing journey. However perfectly we align and balance our chakras today, tomorrow is another day. Our physical body may suffer an infection or accident, or our energetic body may be thrown off balance by an emotional disturbance. Allow yourself this humanity.

When you check in with your chakras, what matters is how they / you are right here and now. There is no need to judge them for being a little off. Just help them back to the right place. And appreciate the empowerment this gives you over your own mental, physical and spiritual state.

Enjoy the upgrade.

Healing our chakras

What improves the state of chakras?

There are lots of practices you can use to improve your chakra health. Either by doing things yourself or by receiving treatment. For example:

- Acupuncture and acupressure work on the meridians to clear blockages causing pain or systemic issues in the body or mind.
- Reiki works at an energetic level to do the same.
- Guided meditations, sometimes using particular colors and sounds also help clear, balance and align chakras
- Specific yoga postures and mudras (hand positions) stimulate particular meridians and points on them
- Ayurvedic guidance recommends certain foods for particular chakras
- Sound healing uses different frequencies that resonate with each chakra to improve their condition

In Part 2 of this book where there is more detail on each chakra you will find some suggestions for how best to nurture each one.

When might chakra healing be useful?

At different points in your life you will feel a need to support different chakras. For example, maybe your heart chakra has become stuck or stagnant as you cope with a relationship breakup or bereavement. Or you spend so much time in your head that all your chakras from the neck down have slowed down and clogged up because you are disconnected from them.

You are also likely to have general tendencies to be stronger or more challenged around different chakras. That may show up as health issues eg a tendency to suffer from tonsillitis or a stiff neck because you are blocked in your throat chakra – caused, for example, from not speaking your truth.

Working with your chakras can help you with both specific problems and wider issues while giving you a chance to balance your physical and emotional systems overall.

It is a delight to tune up your chakras! You are likely to feel more energized, clearer headed, calmer, stronger and healthier. You will find that you have more equanimity – you can go with the flow and see the wider picture. You may notice you don't take things so personally so don't get upset as often.

They are well worth getting to know and supporting – so that they can in turn support you to live the best life you can.

Healing our chakras

I like to keep an overall eye on my chakras through practices such as those described in Part 2 of this book. And I also have some "emergency procedures" that I can use under duress for example on my way to a difficult interaction with someone, or when I need to be especially present and clear.

How: …

Part 2: chakra by chakra guide

How to work with your chakras

In this part of the book we will consider each of the chakras in turn.

There is no fixed way to use this book. You might wish to read all of the information first and then spend some time paying special attention to each chakra. If you do this then I recommend you go in the order of the book (i.e. from root to crown). There's no rush. Spending a couple of days with each chakra will help you get to know it and be able to tap into its energy more easily in future.

Or, you might first do the simple meditation exercise I have included in this section, to help identify where in your body you feel most blocked and start by working with that.

Be aware that your chakras do not have a fixed pattern. While we all have some general tendencies, we are also fluid beings, changing with the seasons or in response to events in our lives.

So, approach this meditation with an open mind and without judgement. It is not a test. You won't get a score for how "good" you are at having chakras, and there is no hierarchy of chakras. They each have different roles and they are all necessary. It is not 'better' to have a strongest crown chakra or a strongest root chakra. We are seeking harmony and integration, so competition has no place here.

Accept what you find. And resist the temptation to compare yourself with others, or to yourself on a different day or during an earlier period in your life.

Whatever state we are in, there will usually be a weakest link. A part of our chakra system that would benefit the most from our loving attention. Seek that out, support it and raise your overall vibration.

Strengthening chakras is not a zero-sum game – there is not a limited amount of power to share out between the chakras. But rather think of the system as just that, an integrated system. The more energy comes in at the bottom – or root chakra – the more energy can make it through our body and up to the crown chakra. We want to maximize the flow and minimize the blockages throughout our integrated whole.

Chakra meditation

(See supporting video on youtube.com/catherineshovlin)

You might have a regular meditation practice, or an occasional practitioner. Or you might never have tried it. All are ok. If you are new to the idea of meditating, I suggest you start by putting aside all your preconceptions. Think of this process as more of a bedtime story. A calming, clarifying time for yourself. A moment of peace and tranquility. If you find you fall asleep halfway through, then accept that your body needed that and try again another time. Maybe in a less comfortable chair! Or not last thing at night.

If you feel that meditation is not for you, then fair enough. You might want to give this 15 minute one a try though just in case you find it gives you any peace of mind.

What doesn't work so well is trying to read the meditation out to yourself while you are also doing it. That activates the wrong parts of our brain for this exercise. So, I suggest you either listen to the audio version on my website - windsofdiscovery.com. Or record yourself reading it then play it back, or have a friend read it aloud to you.

Meditation to get to know your chakras

Find yourself a comfortable position, either seated upright in a chair, cross-legged on the floor or lying down on your back. Whatever position you are in, make sure your spine is straight so your energy can flow freely.

Breathe in deeply - through your nose if you can, or your mouth if you need to. Pause for a second, holding your breath softly, and then exhale through your mouth with a sigh.

Do this a few times and notice how each time you exhale, some tension leaves your body. Inhale… pause… exhale. Inhale… pause… exhale. Inhale… pause… exhale.

How: …Chakra meditation

Now put your attention on your feet. Imagine warm hands are holding them and feel the muscles and joints in your feet relax.

Now imagine those hands holding your calves… and feel them relax.

And resting on the tops of your thighs… so that they can relax.

Feel them hold your right hand, your right forearm, your upper arm… and relax.

Then your left hand, left forearm and left upper arm… and relax.

Feel the warm hands press gently on your shoulders, letting your chest open as you release any tension.

Feel one hand on the back of your head and the other on your forehead. Your head is held securely like this, breathe in deeply though your nose, pause for a second and then exhale gently through your nose.

Still feeling the hands on your forehead and back of your head let's take 3 more long slow breaths in through your nose and out through your nose. Inhale… exhale… inhale… exhale… inhale… exhale.

Then feel the hands move away.

Your whole body is relaxed now.

How: ...Chakra meditation

Start to focus your attention on your root chakra. Right at the bottom of your spine. Imagine a red glow in that part of your body around your tailbone. Feel the warmth. Feel the connection to the earth. Feel gravity pulling your body gently towards the center of the earth.

Imagine that you can breathe in and out through your root chakra. Thank it for taking care of you. For protecting you. For getting you to this point in your life. Give it your loving support.

Now move your awareness to your sacral chakra somewhere around your perineum or pelvic floor. Have a sense of it glowing orange. Feel its energy. Feel its vitality. Feel the power of a vast ocean. Feel the waves gently rocking you.

Imagine that you are breathing in and out through this chakra. Thank it for your appetite. Your appetite for life, for food, for possibility. Give it your loving support.

Move your awareness to your solar plexus chakra just above your navel. Imagine a yellow light pulsing there. Feel its power to move you through your life. Feel the fire in your belly. Your life force. Feel your courage and resilience.

Imagine you are breathing in and out through this chakra. Thank it for its good instincts. Thank it for all your intuition. Thank it for every time your gut feeling was right. Give it your loving support.

Move your awareness to your heart chakra in the center of your chest now. See the soft green light emanating from it.

How: ...Chakra meditation

Feel its healing power. Feel your connection to the people you love. Feel all the love other people have for you. Feel safe. Feel held.

Imagine you are breathing in and out through this chakra. Notice the air flowing in and out of your body.

Thank this chakra for helping you love and be loved. Thank it for the compassion you witness in the world. Thank it for the acts of kindness you give and receive. Give it your loving support.

Move your awareness to your throat chakra. See clear sky-blue light shining there. Feel the beauty of communication and connection with others. Feel the power of speaking your truth. Feel the satisfaction of being heard and understood.

Imagine you are breathing in and out through this chakra. Feel the sky-blue light clear your body.

Thank this chakra for helping you to communicate with the world. Thank it for your self-expression. Thank it for the wide range it gives you, from the gentlest whisper to the mightiest roar. Give it your loving support.

Now move your awareness to your third eye chakra between your eyebrows. Sense a deep blue light glowing there like a beautiful night sky. Feel its depth and infinite possibility. Imagine you have perfect vision into your best future.

How: …Chakra meditation

Imagine you are breathing in and out through this chakra.

Thank this chakra for all that you see physically and mentally. Thank it for the times when you said, "I saw that coming!". Thank it for the times you said, "I see what you mean". Thank it for your vision. And give it your loving support.

Lastly move your awareness to your crown chakra at the top of your head. Sense a violet light shining there. Feel it pulse and glow. Have a sense of great spaciousness. Feel the vastness of the universe. Feel yourself in the story of everything.

Imagine you are breathing in and out through this chakra. You know that you are everything and everything is you. We are all connected in this unifying force. Feel yourself expand to the outer reaches of the universe.

Thank this chakra for all that you can be, and all that humanity can be. For all the growth and expansion that is possible for us. Give it your loving support.

And now pause for a few minutes in this heightened state. Feel your awareness of all of your chakras. Feel the energy in them and flowing between them.

Be gently aware of which ones are strong and which ones want more support. Feel your breath move through your body, gently nurturing all of your chakras. Be aware that you are enhancing your relationship with them.

And now in preparation for ending this meditation let your awareness move from your crown chakra down to your third eye.

Then from there down to your throat chakra, then your heart chakra, your solar plexus chakra, your sacral chakra and finally to your root chakra.

Feel a sense of folding back into yourself. Feel the security and sense of groundedness. Feel the well-being.

Breathe gently for a few moments and then gradually breathe more deeply. Start to feel your fingers and toes. Wiggle them to bring your awareness to the edges of your body. And gently open your eyes.

You might want to take a minute to note anything you observed during this meditation. Which chakras were easier to access and relate to than others?

Note any sense of blockages or tightness or congestion that you came across. This might help you decide where to go first in the next section of the book. Or you might choose to read about all of them and see what resonates for you.

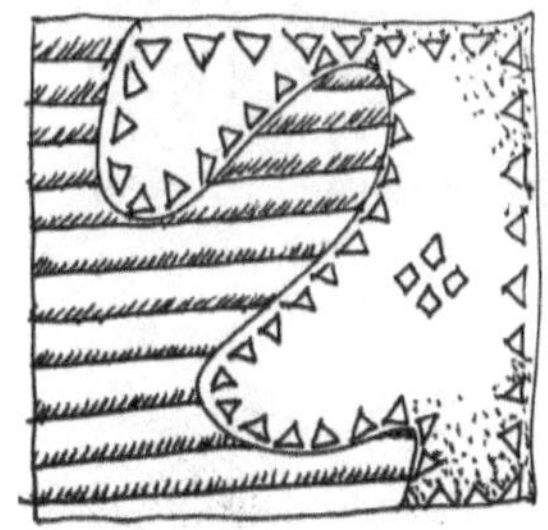

Root chakra

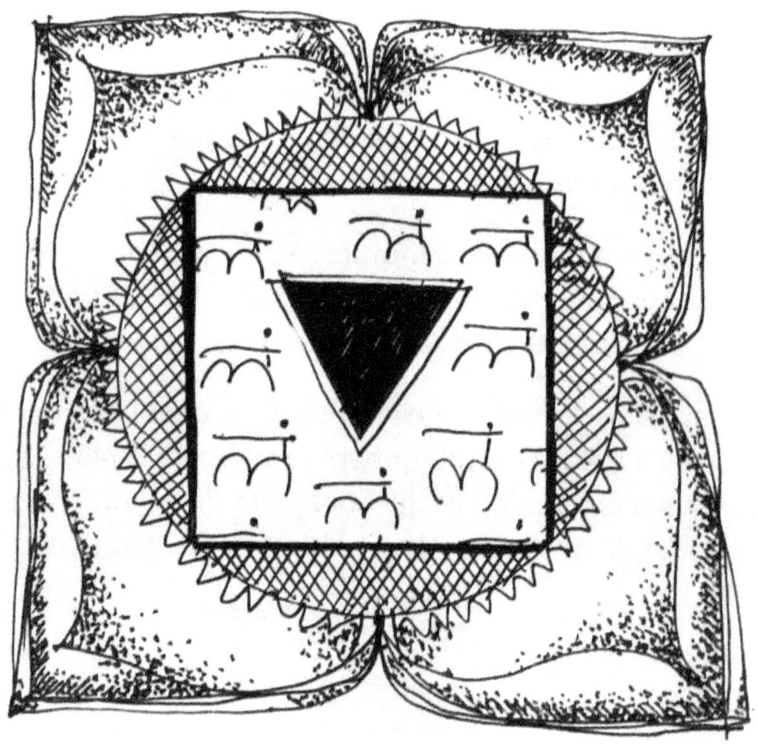

Information about the root chakra

Introduction

Let's start at the foundation, our root chakra or *muladhara* to give it its Sanskrit name. It is located at the base of our spine, the end of your tailbone, near your anus. As with all the chakras, this is an energy center so you can tune into it and feel where it is intuitively. The precise physical location is less important.

As in Maslow's pyramid, this lowest chakra is about survival. Basic instinct. Heat, food, shelter, safety. In modern life that also includes money for most of us - financial security.

Without a firm foundation, nothing else will have the stability it needs to thrive and survive. If we live much of the time in our higher chakras – maybe this is your natural tendency, or maybe your life and work is focused on intellectual or spiritual pursuits - we can lose focus on this important base. Maybe even judge it as beneath us. Too worldly for our higher level of being.

That would be a shame for this rich soil is our root, our connection to the earth. Like a tree that survives a storm because of a deep root structure, being strong in this area will allow our intellectual or spiritual activities to reach even higher levels.

How: …Root chakra

And it is where we root ourselves. In old English, one might refer to someone as 'having bottom'. An instinctive interpretation of the benefits of a strong root chakra. Someone who is grounded and not easily destabilized. Good in a crisis. By the same token, nowadays a horse-rider might be said to have a "good seat".

We also talk about wanting to hunker down, defined by the Cambridge English Dictionary as *"to make yourself comfortable in a place or situation, or to prepare to stay in a place or position for a long time, usually in order to achieve something or for protection"*. This physical and emotional sensation is what we are aiming to achieve with our root chakra work.

Color

The color for this chakra is red - the first color seen by the human eye as we grow from infancy and the first color to be named in the development of most languages.

Red is also the color we physically see first, which in our primal state could have made the difference between life and death after a bad cut or as a poisonous frog or snake appeared. In modern life, spotting and reacting to a red traffic light or quickly finding a fire extinguisher could also keep us alive!

The day after writing this I was watching a skink – a smooth version of a lizard - while eating my Bali. In a matter of minutes, it covered a large area of ground. It moved very fast, only stopping at each red thing. Some were bits of plastic from food packaging, some were leaves, but some were ripe berries which he gobbled up. This focus on red gave the skink a very efficient way of finding food.

Element

The element of the root chakra is, not surprisingly, Earth. All of its qualities of groundedness and being rooted fit with this. With earth we also have earthenware, and the very stable feel of a building made from the earth it stands on.

Earth also represents abundance and nourishment as it provides the means for us to grow and produce food. It is a fundamentally female, or yin element, connected to its role of nourishing and nurturing. Mother Nature.

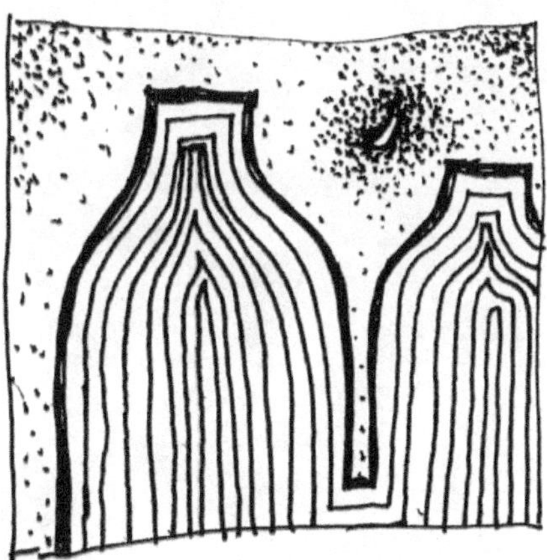

Of course, Earth has its negative aspects too – as seen in the destruction caused by a volcano or earthquake. There is strong power there, which requires our respect. We depend on the Earth for our survival, yet we seem determined to destroy it. That's about as smart as my dog who likes to eat his own bed until he ends up lying on the floor!

Name and symbol

The Sanskrit term for this chakra is *muladhara*. *Mula* meaning root and *adhara* meaning support or base.

Like all the chakras the root chakra has a symbol associated with it. This symbol includes the inverted triangle (representing the earth element) and four lotus petals relating to four key aspects of our sense of self (mind, ego, intellect and consciousness) which we aim to clear and align as we go through our life's journey.

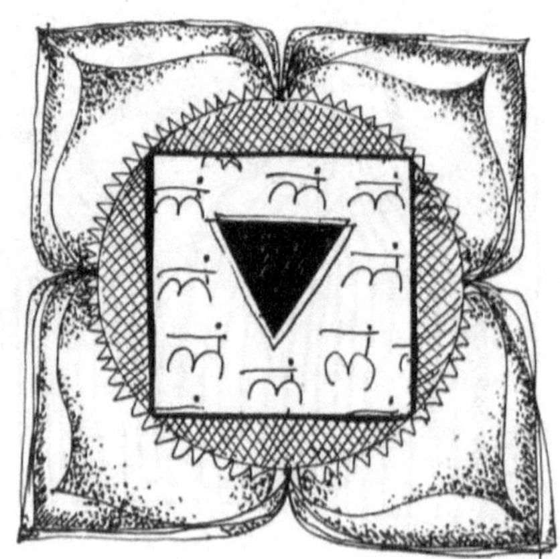

Signs of imbalance in the root chakra

An out of balance root chakra can show up in various ways. We have many everyday expressions invoking this part of our body – often relating to extreme fear.

Physical signs

If you have an imbalance or blockage in this chakra you might experience lower back problems. Of course, there may be physical reasons for this too, such as working with small children, but the fact that some of us are affected by something while others are not is an indicator that the chakras are also playing a role.

An imbalance in this chakra can also be indicated by fatigue or weight gain associated with poor elimination or constipation.

Emotional and psychological signs

An underactive or blocked root chakra can show up as a lack of self-love or an inability to have clear boundaries. As a consequence, you might find yourself being a martyr to other people's needs, a bit of a doormat or even having a victim mentality. You may also experience a lot of fear and anger

Psychologically you may feel that life doesn't support you. That everything is always a struggle. That it's just not fair. If your root chakra is blocked or out of balance, you may have

How: …Root chakra

a strong need to control as much as you can to try to push away the fear that you feel.

Supporting your root chakra

By clearing and balancing this chakra you can experience an increased sense of self, of knowing who you are. You can welcome a feeling of acceptance of yourself exactly as you are. You could move to a place where you value yourself and manage your boundaries appropriately for your own protection.

Here are some techniques that might appeal. There are no hard and fast rules here. Use your intuition and work with whatever feels right for you. You can try one thing or several. See what is best aligned with your lifestyle and preferences. The more interested you are in the action the more likely it is to help.

Yoga support

(See supporting video on youtube.com/catherineshovlin)

Raise awareness of root chakra

.

Sit in a comfortable cross-legged position (easy pose) on the floor if you can, or on a chair if you need to. You may want

How: …Root chakra

to put a folded towel under your tailbone to help your spine find its natural curve

Put your attention on your root chakra. Rock back and forth slightly, tilting your pelvis as you do so, moving from your sit-bones to your tailbone and back. Feel the energy in that part of your body and visualize it glowing red.

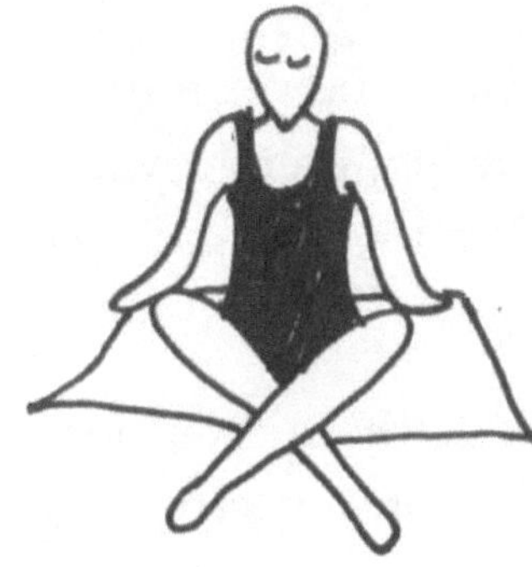

When we are seated, our root chakra is grounded, connected to the earth. Imagine that you are drawing up energy from the core of the earth. Pulling it into your body and warming the base of your spine.

Now with your hands on your knees, rock your pelvis back slightly, hollowing your belly as you exhale. Then tilt it forward, so your belly is moving towards your thighs. Lead the movement with your heart, not your head, and inhale.

Keep repeating this motion for a minute. Exhaling as you hollow and tilt back, inhaling as you move forward. Imagine the inhalation is coming up through your root chakra and bringing all the strength and stability of the earth into your body. As you exhale, feel that you are releasing all that you no longer need into the earth, knowing that it can process whatever you give it.

Next, staying in this seated position, with your hands on your knees, rotate your body in a clockwise direction. Try to keep your legs and your head in the same place, really feel the movement in your torso – your ribcage and hips.

Inhale as you move to the right then back and open up your body, exhale as you move round to the left, then forwards. Do 5 rotations in that direction and then reverse and do 5 in the other direction.

Really feel your groundedness as you do these rotations. Keep both sit-bones in contact with the chair or ground at all times.

Activate root chakra

Now, if you can, sit in a kneeling position (thunderbolt) with your bottom on your heels. Feel free to use a cushion on your heels and/or a blanket under your ankles or knees if you feel any discomfort. If your knees cannot take this position, then sit on a chair.

If you can, clasp your hands behind your back with your arms straight. Or hold your opposite elbows, also behind your back. If you cannot do either of those then put your hands on your hips.

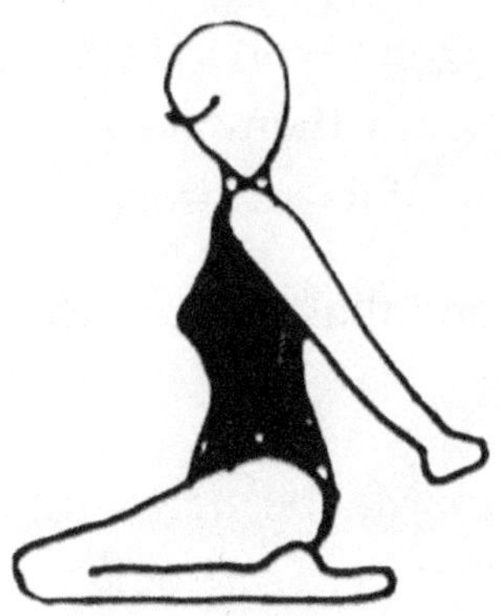

 Inhale and look up to the sky, exhale and fold forwards as far as is comfortable for you. Don't strain your back, the important thing is to feel the movement in your root chakra, it doesn't matter how far you bend. Feel the movement as your belly moving towards your feet, not towards your knees.

Inhale and look up, exhale and fold forward again. Repeat this for about a minute.

Root lock

To finish, it can give great support to your digestive system if you exercise the sphincter muscles around your anus.

There are two rings of muscle, one at the exit to control release (or not!) of stool and one internally. It is the external one that we can control consciously.

How: …Root chakra

Sit or lie in a comfortable position. Take a deep inhale, then as you exhale, contract this muscle. Don't worry if it is hard to isolate at first. If you do this every day then you will quickly develop a more precise sense of its location.

Release and contract it 10 times. Then inhale and pause, holding the breath.

Repeat this as many times as you can. Maybe start with 20 (two rounds) and then build up over time. The yogis recommend 200 contractions per day. I usually do 100 and have noticed that it gets easier over time. Once you get the feel for it, this is something you can easily do while watching TV or in the car or the bus.

There are many things we cannot control in life but having good control over your continence helps with self-respect as well as having obvious physical benefits.

Supporting activities

- Walk, especially barefoot and especially in nature. Notice your connection to the earth with each footfall
- Stamp the ground to release excess emotion
- Sit on the ground and beat a drum – or wooden box – with your hands
- Write a fear inventory of all the things you fear. Use the format "I fear … because …". Then read it out loud to a friend, or the dog or a tree. Accept that you have these fears. Now tear up the paper into small pieces and throw it away (responsibly of course).

- Use the color red. I'm a big fan of red knickers (underpants) for the sense of safety and strength they give. If you want to strengthen your energy in this chakra you might use a red cloth over a lamp to fill the room with red light or adjust your LED lighting to red if you have that option. Try doing that for half an hour while you meditate on your root chakra or do the yoga moves suggested above.

Sound support

Use middle C on the Western scale, or a note low in your range that feels natural to you, to hum or chant to attune this chakra. Feel the sound reverberate in that part of your body, around about your anus and the bottom of your tailbone. You can chant LAM (pronounced lormm) with each long exhale.

You can also find chakra specific music on YouTube (search *Meditative Mind* for a good selection) or Spotify. Search for *muladhara* or root chakra. Let it play in the background while you are working or travelling for a few days and see if it starts to shift your perceptions and sense of self.

Nutritional support

Grounding food that aligns with your root chakra energy includes root vegetables (carrots, sweet potatoes, parsnips, beetroot, turnips), spices from roots (eg garlic, ginger, turmeric) as well as red foods like paprika and pepper. Food

How: …Root chakra

rich in protein like tofu, eggs, nuts, meat if you eat it, red beans and red lentils are also helpful.

Recipe for earthy soup

Try making this rich, comforting soup to love up your root chakra.

Ingredients

- 1 tbsp olive oil
- 1 onion, chopped
- 2 garlic cloves, chopped or grated
- 1 nub of ginger, finely chopped
- Spices: ½ tsp ground cumin, ½ tsp ground coriander, ½ tsp ground turmeric, salt and pepper to taste
- 1 large sweet potato, chopped into ½ cm cubes
- 1 red pepper, chopped into ½ cm cubes
- 2 carrots, chopped into ½ cm cubes
- 1 cube or pack of vegetable stock dissolved in 3 cups of hot water
- 1 cup of red lentils
- ½ cup of mixed nuts, dry roasted and chopped
- A few chives

Instructions

1. Heat the oil in a large heavy bottomed saucepan over a low heat
2. Gently fry the onion, garlic and ginger for 5-10 mins till soft

3. Add the spices and fry for one more minute
4. Add the carrots, sweet potato and pepper and cook for a minute or two, stirring to coat the vegetables with the oil and spice mixture
5. Add the vegetable stock
6. Add the lentils.
7. Turn the heat down and leave to simmer for 15 mins or until the lentils are soft. Stir occasionally and add more water if necessary.
8. You may prefer to have the soup as it is or use a blender for a creamy consistency.
9. Top with a sprinkle of nuts and chopped chives

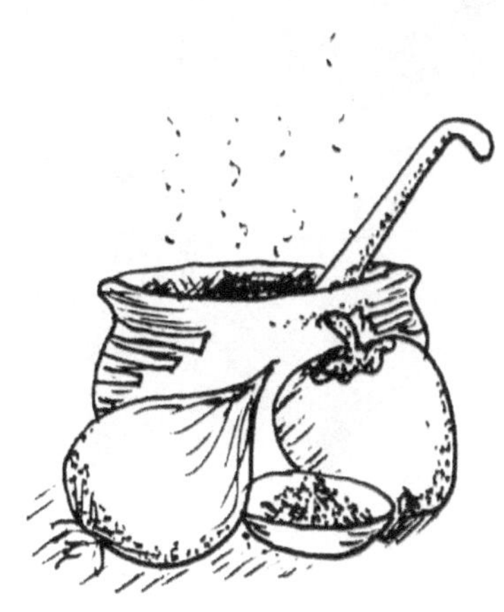

Sacral chakra

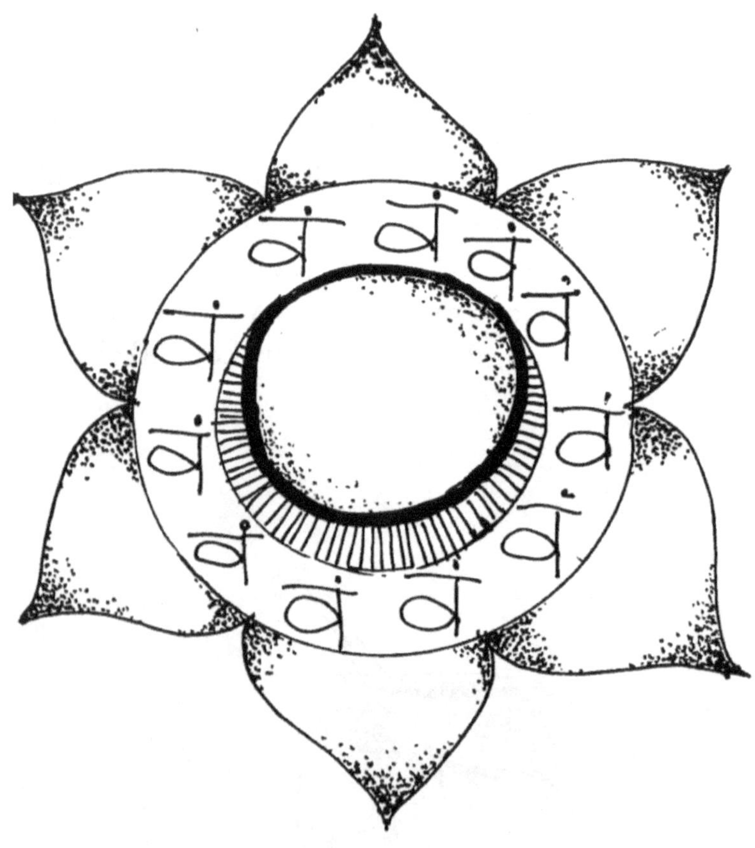

Information about the sacral chakra

Introduction

The sacral chakra is located close to the root chakra but a little higher. Feel for the top of your pubic bone and imagine a point deep inside you at about that level. Inside the vagina, near the cervix for women, and up from the perineum in men.

Physically this chakra is associated with the reproductive organs in both men and women. It is also closely connected to the lymphatic system – our own drainage system to clear the body of unwanted by-products of cellular activity.

It is closely connected with feelings and sensations. Including creativity and the good feelings derived from pleasurable activities to do with sensual or other physical sensations like eating delicious food, the feel of silk or a soft breeze on your skin.

You might call this the well-being chakra. Nurture it by nurturing yourself. And pay attention to it when it's crying out for help.

Color

The color for the sacral chakra is orange. With all its warmth and energy, its fire.

When we talk about zest for life, maybe we are deriving that from the zest of an orange – the zing and energy of orange oil. Flick through any cookery book and you will notice how strongly the color orange features – baked goods, orange vegetables, golden fried food.

Physiologically the color orange stimulates appetite and that makes perfect sense for this chakra. Notice if this color makes you feel uncomfortable. That could be an indication that you are suppressing your appetites. A common behavior, especially for women, in a world that values slimness and which historically has discouraged women from expressing their desires.

Element

The element associated with this chakra is water. That life-giving force that makes up around 60% of our bodies and without which life is not possible.

It is unusual for a molecule which doesn't include carbon to be liquid under what we consider to be normal conditions (the temperatures and pressures we happily live in). Thank goodness it is!

From a scientific point of view, water is a very special molecule with a high specific heat capacity. It provides temperature stability on the earth thanks to its remarkably high boiling point (considering its molecular weight).

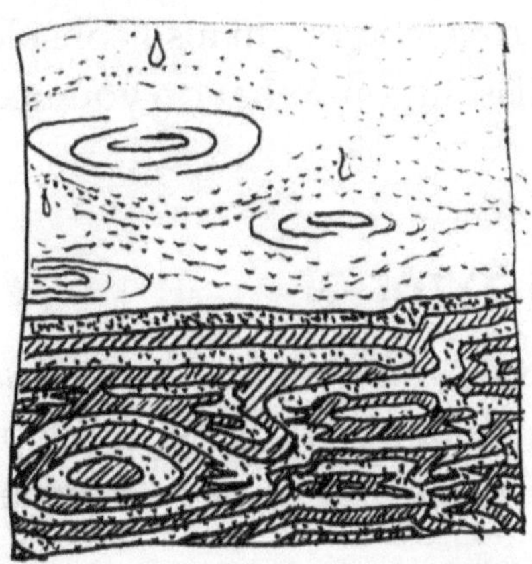

It has a wide temperature range as a liquid, between being a solid (freezing as ice at 0 degrees Celsius) and being a gas (changing to water vapor at 100 degrees Celsius). This means that lots of life forms can live in it under a good range of temperature conditions without suddenly finding the water they are in, or that is in them, freezing or vaporizing. Within our bodies, water plays a similar role. Sweating to cool us and holding body temperature stable when the atmosphere around us is cold.

Even when water does freeze over, in a lake or the sea for example, the ice on the surface forms a buffer zone so that the rest of the water can remain liquid and life can continue. How can you use the life-giving properties of this chakra to serve you? Where do you seek more stability and protection in your life?

Water also has the special property of being able to dissolve a wide range of substances. I won't go into the chemistry of this – those who are interested can easily research it - but in metaphysical terms, you might also consider this chakra as important for dissolution. What do you need to dissolve in your life?

Name and Symbol

The sacral chakra is known as *Svadhishthana* in Sanskrit. *Svadhi* meaning self and *shthana* meaning place. It relates to our place in the world, our sense of aliveness.

This shows up in our lives as our appetites, our zest for life (or lack of it if this chakra is blocked or out of kilter).

The ancient symbol for this chakra has the same circle that is the basis for all of the chakras, signifying our unity and eternity. In the center it has another circle positioned to create a crescent moon on the bottom rim.

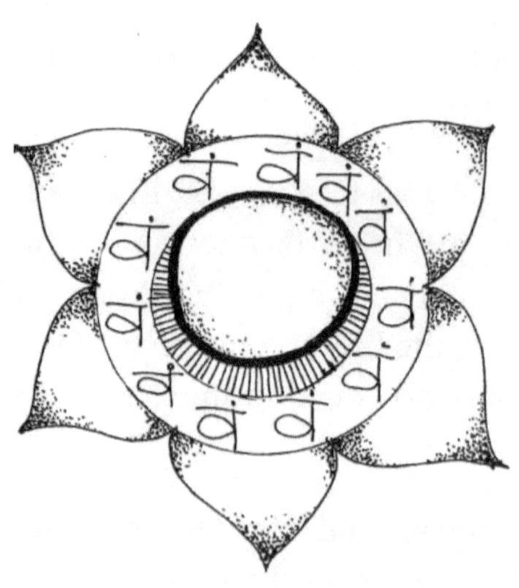

How: ...Sacral chakra

The moon - and the tides that it creates in the oceans and in the waters within us - is a reminder of the cycles of life. Monthly cycles in women, that continue even after menopause, the circles of life and death, or day and night.

We are all subjected to changes due to external circumstances, throughout our lives. The weather, political changes, bereavements and redundancies. As the Buddhists say, we cannot avoid the first arrow of unwanted events, but we can avoid the second arrow by choosing how we will react. Will we suffer, dwell on issues, fret? Or will we accept and learn and adjust?

The same might be said of the changes in our bodies as we progress though our lives. Being a teenager, suffering from PMS, experiencing pregnancy, noticing how our bodies change as we age and our metabolisms shift, going grey or bald, health conditions, menopause, terminal illness. We cannot avoid experiencing some or all of these things yet often we resist them. Are you accepting the changes in your life with good grace? Or fighting them tooth and nail?

Signs of imbalance in the sacral chakra

Physical signs

An imbalance in this area can affect the sexual organs in this region. So, it might show up as menstrual difficulties, challenges in fertility, ovarian cysts or prostrate issues –

depending on what body parts you have. Regardless of your gender you may experience a drop in libido.

Also in this region we have the bladder and kidneys, governed by this chakra. Physical consequences of an imbalance in the sacral chakra can include NSU (non-specific urethritis), kidney stones and the lower back pain associated with the kidneys.

Emotional and Psychological signs

Emotional challenges arising if we need to boost this chakra include anger, jealousy or false pride. We can work on strengthening or balancing this chakra to free ourselves from the heavy toll of these emotions.

Psychologically, if this chakra is out of balance, we may deny ourselves simple pleasures. Feeling some sense of nobility in denying our appetites. This is a choice that any of us are free to make in life of course, but it might be worth taking a moment to consider your motives. Where is this self-denial coming from? Is it your own, or something you have picked up from parents, teachers or people you wish to impress? Is it giving you what you really want, or might this be a time to accept the change in season and shift to a different way of life?

You may also be out of balance in the opposite direction and find yourself over-reacting, being a bit of a drama queen, or feeling overwhelmed. For women this can be exacerbated by hormonal changes such as puberty, menstruation, pregnancy or menopause. Not surprising as these are all related to the reproductive organs closely connected to this chakra.

You may find that you are more sensitive than usual, more prone to taking things personally and assuming every action from other people is specifically designed to hurt you.

Another manifestation is finding yourself unable to bear other people's emotions and withdrawing to find peace in your solitude.

If you are naturally creative, there might be times when the creative storm feels too much. This is a good reminder to balance your sacral chakra for a healthy, sustainable level of creativity.

Supporting your sacral chakra

Yoga support

(See supporting video on youtube.com/catherineshovlin)

As this chakra is physically close to the root chakra, many of the same movements will help it. Here are also some more flowing (water like) movements that you might want to try to improve balance in your sacral chakra.

Kali power flow

Kali is a powerful goddess, clearing out what is not needed.

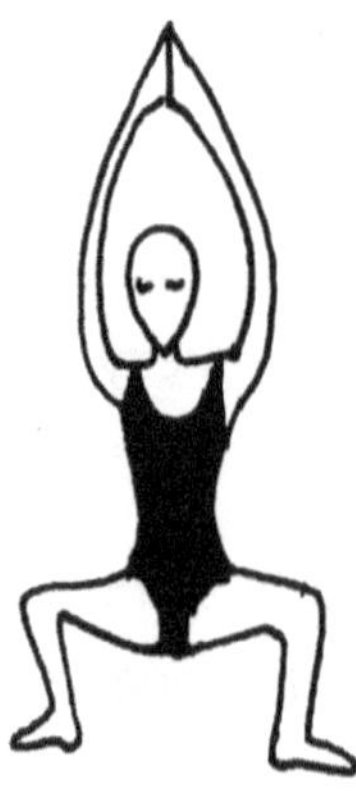

Start standing with feet about a leg's length apart. Bend your knees so you are in a powerful squat with your knees over your feet (check you can still see your toes, so you don't put too much strain on your knees. If you can't go down very far then do what you can).

Stretch your arms out parallel to the floor and then as you inhale, slowly straighten your legs and raise your arms until your palms touch above your head.

Exhale and bend your legs again, lowering your arms until they are parallel to the floor.

Inhale and straighten your legs, lifting your arms.

Exhale and bend your legs, lowering your arms.

Repeat this for about one minute, feeling the power in your lower belly and knowing that you have the strength to clear what is no longer needed from your life.

How: ...Sacral chakra

Imagine Kali and the element of water sluicing out what is
no longer required leaving you cleansed and ready for your
next step.

Up and down flowing dog

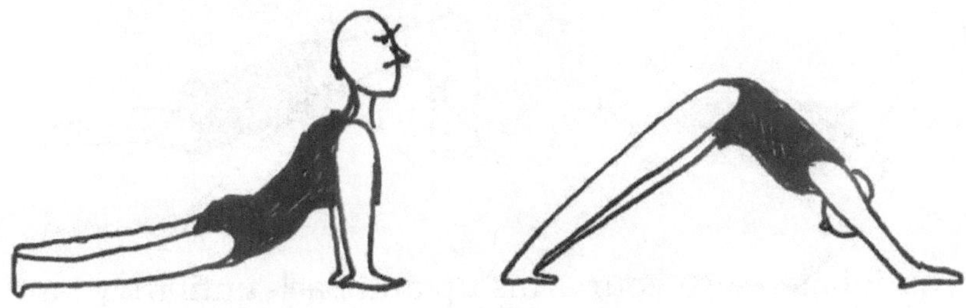

Now placing both hands on the floor in front of you, step
your feet back into downward dog.

Check your shoulders are relaxed and away from the ears.
Keep your legs bent if that feels better for you. Feel the lift in
your pelvis as though someone was standing behind you
with their hands under your hip bones pulling you
upwards.

As you inhale shift your hips down to the floor and raise
your head and chest to upward dog.

Then exhale back to downward dog.

Repeat this short sequence 5 times in total, or more if you
feel like it. Keep the movement as flowing as you can, work
with your breath and sense the flow stimulating your
sacrum and sacral chakra.

Water flowing under the Bridge

Lie on your back and move your feet so they are flat on the floor, as close to your buttocks as you can comfortably manage. Rest your hands by your sides.

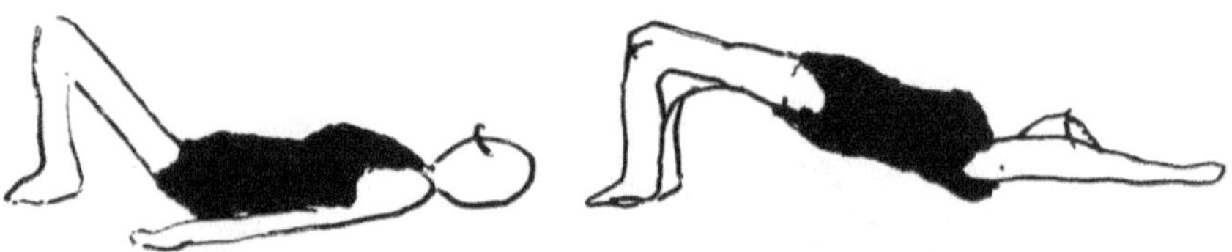

As you inhale, raise your arms up and back until they land on the floor behind you, while at the same time, you raise your hips. Imagine the cleansing waters flowing under the bridge you have made.

As you exhale, curl your spine back down, from the neck, vertebra by vertebra as you simultaneously bring your arms up and over to land back at your sides at the same time as your bottom arrives back on the floor at the end of your exhale.

Repeat this flowing movement for about a minute.

Get your juices flowing

Finish with another contraction exercise, this time of the perineum and, for women, the vagina around the cervix. If you have a jade egg you can use this to further refine your practice and stimulate reflexology points in your vagina.

How: ...Sacral chakra

Take a deep inhale and then exhale as you pull the muscles in your pelvic floor and vagina up as though you were drawing them towards your naval. Contract and release these muscles ten times with your breath held out.

Inhale and exhale then do another round of ten contractions.

As with the root chakra, start by doing 20 of these – two rounds - and then see how you can build up your capacity to 100 or even 200 per day.

You might notice how this triggers some emotional response in you. Maybe there is a lot of sadness in this part of your body, say from a miscarriage, traumatic birth or lack of sexual satisfaction. Be tender with yourself and know that you are building strength and resilience in this aspect of your being.

A healthy sexuality is important for all of us, whatever life stage we are at. And a strong pelvic floor has a lot of other benefits too for your health and well-being.

Do these exercises with kindness and a good heart, just do as much as feels right for you and notice how gradually it is easier.

Supporting activities

Nurture this chakra with sensual activities that make you feel good.

How: …Sacral chakra

Be a water baby

Being in water is the natural element for this chakra. Take a swim if that works for you – ideally outdoors in natural water with the sky overhead and the sound of birds singing.

Even better if you can be somewhere you feel comfortable swimming naked. Notice the feel of the water on your skin and relish it.

Or run yourself a beautiful warm bath with essential oils, candles and your favorite music. Maybe even sprinkle a few rose petals onto the water for that extra sense of luxury.

Sensual pleasures

Loving, delicious sex or self-pleasuring is an obvious option for this chakra.

I realize that some of you may have grown up in a culture where these activities were viewed as shameful or bad in some ways. That is unfortunate, because a healthy sexuality is a supportive component of everybody's well-being. In whatever form that takes for you. So, experiment with allowing yourself to have sexual needs and reactions. Like other aspects of our persona, this can atrophy if it is neglected. Sometimes you may have to give yourself a pep talk! But, especially for women, it can be something that benefits from a regular practice – however you achieve that.

Whether you are alone or with a partner for this activity, be fully present. Honor your body and your responses. Take

How: ...Sacral chakra

your time and really notice how each pleasurable movement makes you feel – and find the boldness in yourself to suggest adjustments to your partner to maximize your pleasure. Bear in mind that women have twice as many nerve endings per square millimeter in this area than men do. So, you may need to do some coaching to help your partner understand the difference.

The more you notice about your own body and what works for it, the more reaction you will be able to enjoy.

Let nature heal you

A walk out in nature is a tonic on so many levels. Take your time. This is not about fitness, it's about well-being.

Notice the bird song, the colors of the plants and the depth of the landscape. What can you hear? How many shades of green can you see?

Breathe in the beauty of the place and give it your appreciation. Maybe take a few moments to sit still in a good spot and take it all in.

If taking pictures or sketching helps you to be fully present, then try that.

A feast for the senses

Prepare a special meal for yourself or to share with loved ones. Even if you are on your own, take care to make it a beautiful experience.

How: ...Sacral chakra

Consider how you want the table to look, the music you want to hear, the kind of lighting that will make you feel good. Enjoy choosing some of your favorite food, shopping for ingredients that are as natural as possible and cooking it with love.

When you come to enjoy your meal, savor every mouthful. Be thankful that you can do this for yourself, that the earth provides us with such a magnificent range of foodstuffs and flavors. Appreciate whoever gave you the recipes – your grandmother or the internet! Notice the taste and texture of the food and the nourishment it is giving you.

Paying attention in this way increases the pleasure of food – and as a bonus, it also increases its nutritional value because you are triggering your digestive system to be ready for it.

Dance like nobody's watching

If you can be free from self-consciousness when dancing with others, then that's great. Find the venues and events that suit you best.

And if not, or if the opportunity doesn't arise, then dancing alone can also be liberating.

Find music that inspires you and dance your most sensuous dance. Enjoy moving your body without any concern for what anyone else might think. Dance your wild dance. The way you would dance if nothing was stopping you.

How: ...Sacral chakra

Forget all the rules, though if you want some ideas, you may want to use something like belly dancing, ecstatic dance or 5 Rhythms to get you started.

Sound support

You can make a playlist for yourself of the songs that make you feel good. It's different for everyone and may reflect special memories or just be a rhythm that you feel vibrating in this chakra.

There are lots of soundtracks on YouTube for the sacral chakra, find one you feel resonates with you and lie back and enjoy.

You can also hum or chant to attune this chakra. The Sanskrit sound for the sacral chakra is VAM (pronounced vomm) and the note on the Western scale is D.

Nutritional support

Foods that work well for this chakra include oily fish such as sardines, mackerel or cod (you may prefer to take this as a fish oil supplement). Salmon is perfect because its orange color also resonates with this chakra. The strong relationship fish have with water is a good fit for the sacral chakra.

The luscious sensual pleasure of mangoes, passion fruit and other tropical fruit is a delight for this chakra. Enjoy their sweet succulence, a feast for the senses. Smell their fragrance, enjoy their abundant appearance, feel their soft

How: ...Sacral chakra

juiciness and of course taste them, allowing them to nourish your body with their rich cocktail of vitamins and minerals.

Nowadays coconut is more and more prevalent, especially in vegan cooking. This too is good protection for the sacral chakra.

Recipe for Sensual Salad

Salad doesn't need to be worthy or dull! Enjoy creating this radiant mixture of ingredients to delight your second chakra.

Ingredients

- Tropical fruit - see what's in your local market, choose from mango, papaya, pineapple, banana, coconut and so on. Go for what feels right for you, your body knows what it needs. Fresh is much better than canned or frozen for a direct connection with the fruit, but sometimes we have to be pragmatic!
- Salmon fillet – go for super fresh and the best quality so you can eat it raw.
- Mild baby salad leaves. Save stronger flavors like rocket (rucola) for your solar plexus chakra.
- A handful of seeds
- Olive or flaxseed oil, apple cider vinegar, soy sauce or lemon juice for dressing if required.

Instructions

1. Heat a medium sized frying pan on medium-high and dry roast the seeds

2. Slice the salmon into 3-5mm pieces, sashimi style. If you don't like the idea of raw salmon, flash fry it in a little olive oil.
3. Prepare the fruit, peeling and cutting it into bite sized pieces
4. Pile your plate with green leaves, then add the tropical fruit and top with the fish and the seeds.
5. Dress and season as required.
6. Eat with pleasure, savoring each mouthful and noticing the combination of tastes and textures.

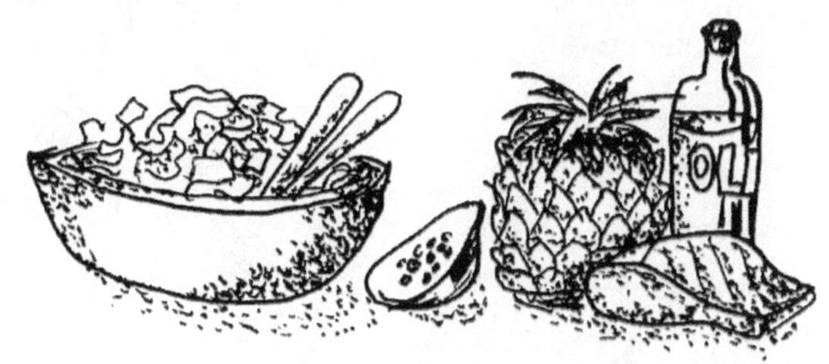

Solar plexus chakra

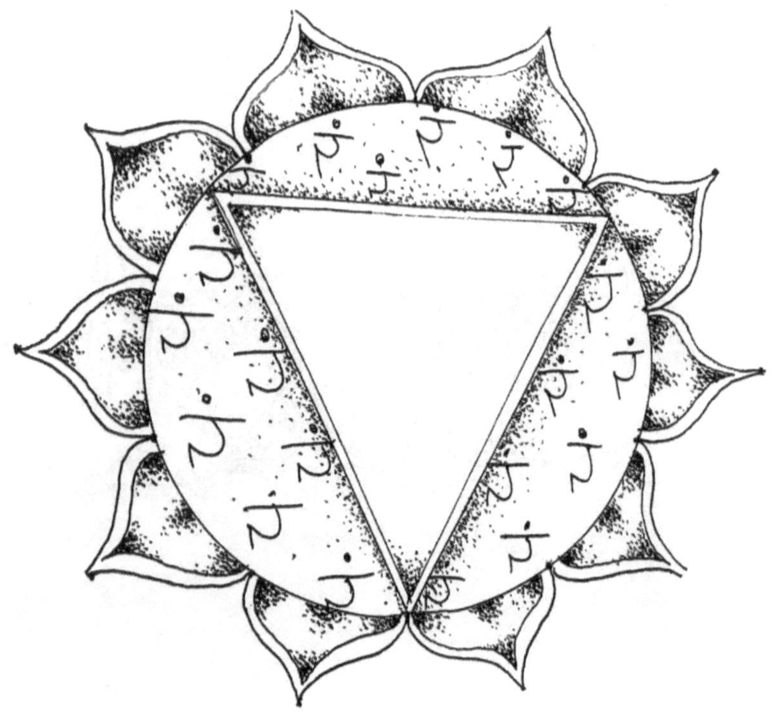

Information about the solar plexus chakra

Introduction

The solar plexus chakra, the seat of our power, is located above your navel, round about the bottom of the rib cage at the front. Long associated with power and a sense of self in Eastern traditions, it is now also recognized by Western medicine as holding a cluster of neurons (like brain cells). So much so, that neuroscientists are referring to it as the abdominal brain.

Its name, the solar plexus, derives in part from the radial connections it has with many of the organs in this part of the body – like the rays of the sun.

The solar plexus chakra is the center of our sense of self and the place we hold in the world. As in "knowing your place". Massage or reflexology techniques that focus on this spot often induce a feeling of 'coming home'. Coming home to yourself. To your true nature, independent of the desires and expectations of the world, society and those close to us.

This integrity and authenticity to our true self is an important aspect of a conscious life. We may talk of "feeling sick to the stomach" when asked to do something which compromises our values. Or being "unable to stomach" something which we find unacceptable.

This chakra is also the basis for our presence – the way we are in the room or the world as we move through it. When

How: …Solar plexus chakra

you are about to embark on an important conversation, or a public speech or performance, it is well worth spending a moment attuning to this chakra so it can support you in your endeavors. Allowing your true strengths to shine.

Color

The solar plexus chakra resonates with the color yellow - also clearly connected to the sun. In popular culture it is the color of optimism and cheerfulness – yet also of cowardice ("yellow belly").

In fact the color yellow does have the physiological effect on us of stimulating the endocrine system and therefore increasing our emotional response. It tends to amplify our mood – so if you're feeling great then that's a good day for a yellow shirt, but not if you feel depression creeping up on you. It increases integrity as it makes you more true to your emotions – but that may not always be convenient.

This chakra is therefore associated with our metabolism as well as our drive, our impetus to get things done here on earth.

Element

The solar plexus chakra is associated with the element of fire – again that makes sense with the sun connotation. It is associated with passionate creativity and zeal "she was on fire!". It is a powerful element which consumes but also warms. Essential to survival, keeping away enemies for our ancestors, making our food easier to digest and keeping us warm.

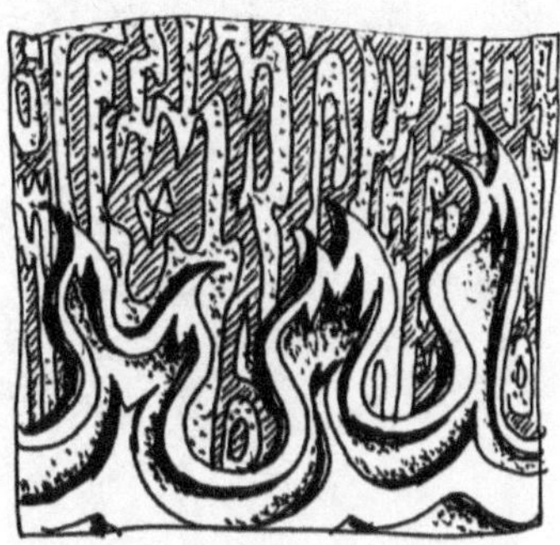

Name and Symbol

The Sanskrit name for the solar plexus chakra is *manipura*, holding the meanings of jewel (*mani*) and place (*pura*). It is both precious and key to our position, our stance.

The inverted triangle in the center of symbol for the solar plexus chakra relates to attraction and emission of energy. Our interchange with the world. You have probably seen power dances performed by indigenous cultures before battle (or a game of rugby!). They work on this area and power it up. This is both for their own resolve and strength in the contest, and also to project their power so that the opposition might think twice about engaging with them.

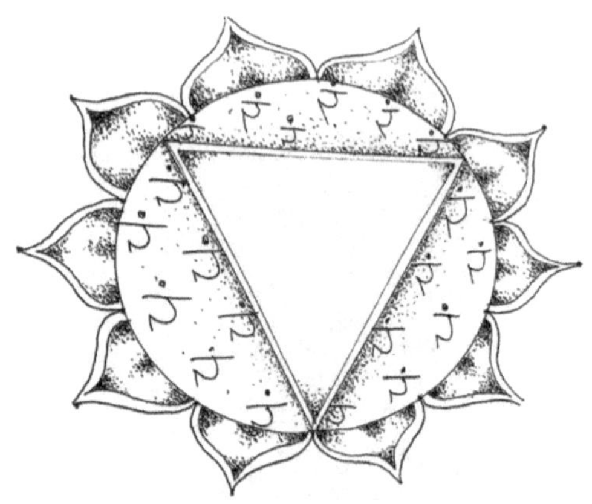

You will see that there are 10 lotus flower petals around the outside of this chakra. These are interpreted in different ways as either the 10 pranas, or energies, that we have flowing through us, or the ten vices that can be stumbling blocks to the free flow of our energy and spirit. Either way it is a good reminder of our mortal selves and how we can pay attention to the way we are in the world.

Signs of imbalance in the solar plexus chakra

Physical signs

Because of its location, this chakra is connected to all of the major organs in the belly. The kidneys, liver, stomach and bowels, as well as having a key relationship with the pancreas – best known in the case of diabetes for insulin production, but also important for all of us in converting our food into energy.

As well as affecting our general nutrition levels and sense of well-being, digestive problems associated with this chakra can in turn affect conditions like diabetes and arthritis. We may suffer from indigestion, bloating or gas if this chakra is blocked. More ongoing problems might result in stomach ulcers or IBS (irritable bowel syndrome).

Emotional and Psychological signs

Emotionally, because it plays a key role in our sense of self, this chakra relates to our self-esteem, self-confidence and capacity to feel good about our circumstances – this can be surprisingly independent from what our circumstances are. We all know of people who seem to have everything and yet are miserable while I have also worked with people during famine, in refugee camps and approaching death, who can be joyful.

How: …Solar plexus chakra

A poor sense of self and low self-esteem is associated with depression and anxiety. A lack of self-confidence or self-belief may in turn lead to co-dependency and a susceptibility to addictive behaviors.

Supporting your solar plexus chakra

Yoga support

(See supporting video on youtube.com/catherineshovlin)

You may well pay attention to this area of your body at the gym, doing ab work to try to improve the appearance of your belly. In yoga terms, we look not so much at hardening muscles as toning them. The internal abdominal muscle structure is also important as the support system for our organs, holding everything in an optimal position for its function.

Here are some simple yoga moves that will awaken, support and balance the solar plexus chakra, keeping its fire burning – while maintaining muscle length and flexibility.

Fire up!

Fire breath is a yogic breathing method that uses the diaphragm to expel air. It gives a good work out to our internal organs and a massage to this area. It is a fast breath.

To start with stand with feet hip width apart, knees slightly bent and hands on thighs, thumbs to the center.

Breathe in and then exhale sharply with a *hah!* sound as you pull your diaphragm inwards and upwards to push out the air. Your inhalation will come naturally as you release the pull and allow the air to flow back into your lungs. Now repeat this quickly (about twice per second). Do a round of ten breaths like this followed by a pause for a regular breath. Try 2 or 3 rounds the first time and then gradually over the coming days, work up to 10 rounds.

Fire Boat

Now go onto the floor and sit with your legs in front of you. There are different levels of this pose depending on what feels comfortable for you today. It is not important how advanced the pose is, it is important that it is right for you.

That might not be the same level as was right for you last week or ten years ago. Listen to your body and do what feels like it is working your belly without putting undue strain on your lower back.

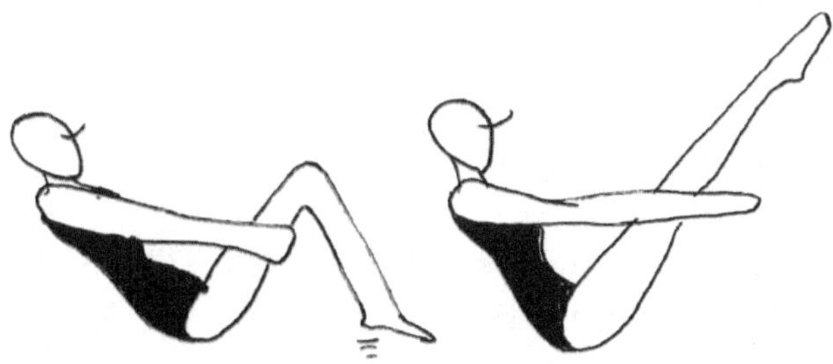

How: ...Solar plexus chakra

For the first level, bend your knees, wrap your arms under your thighs and lift your feet a little off the floor. You will find that there is a point on your sacrum (tail bone) where you can balance in this position - you may have to rock back and forth a little to find the sweet spot.

If this is feels very easy for you then for the second level straighten your legs and point your feet towards the sky.

For the third level, and for more challenge, straighten your arms too.

Once you are in the right position for you today, do 3 rounds of fire breath here (10 breaths per round).

Fire Twist

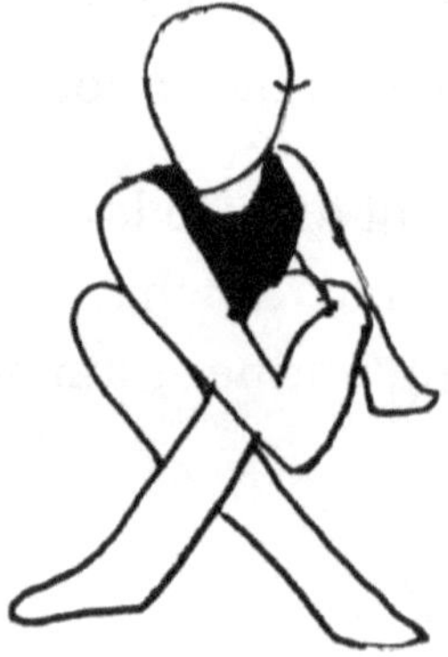

This seated twist will stimulate digestion.

Sit on the floor in cross legged pose and prepare to twist first to the right. Put your right hand behind you on the floor for support and lift up in your spine and lower ribs as you

How: …Solar plexus chakra

inhale. As you exhale, twist to the right, bringing your left arm around the outside of your right knee. Keep your spine as upright as possible and relax your face and shoulders.

Relax in the position for 5 slow breaths then release and repeat on the other side.

Fire Child

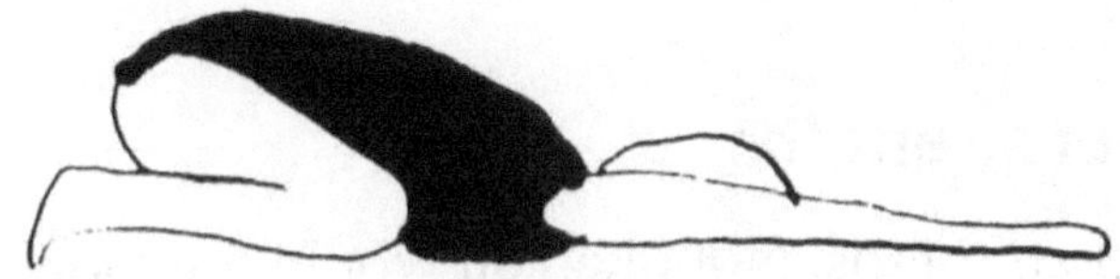

Let's finish this sequence by coming into child's pose.

Kneel on the floor then fold forward over your knees aiming to place your forehead on the floor.

Use a cushion between ankles and hips if that feels more comfortable and a folded under your knees and/or under the fronts of your ankles if necessary.

You may also wish to have a cushion or block if your forehead is not reaching the floor… it is soothing to have this gentle pressure on your forehead. Or you can make fists of your hands to provide support.

Stay here for a minute or two, knowing that this gentle, relaxed pose is still helping you, stimulating the nerves around the solar plexus and helping with bloating or

How: …Solar plexus chakra

indigestion. Don't worry if it has an immediate effect on any trapped gas – this is completely normal and healthy.

Supporting activities

Support your solar plexus chakra with activities that remind you of who you are and why you matter. That strengthen your sense of self, giving you a good foundation to reach out to others.

Strengthen your strengths

Make a list of your strengths. Not like you would for a job application but the things about yourself that you value. Think of specific moments in your life when you have felt that you really came through, standing up for yourself or for others, showing leadership, being present. Your moments of magnificence.

They don't need to be winning the Olympics. It might for instance be a moment when your child got hurt and you were heroic in your compassion. Or tension was building between other people and you stepped in and diffused it. Or you saw injustice and spoke up.

This isn't a time for modesty, this is a time for honesty and clarity. However insignificant a strength may seem to you… you can own it.

Bear in mind that the things we are good at seem easy to us. So, you might need the mirror of a trusted friend to point

How: …Solar plexus chakra

out your strengths to you. Watch out for self-deprecating responses like "Oh that was nothing, anybody would have done the same thing". Just breathe and say thank you.

If all else fails think of ways other people cannot or choose not to do things that seem obvious to you (mental arithmetic, knitting, cooking, listening…). That is a clue that you probably have skill in this area.

Embodiment

Take up a martial art or do some embodiment training to reconnect your sense of self with your body. In our modern world we can easily become disassociated and live primarily in our heads. These practices will bring you into the here and now.

If you don't relate to the energy levels of something like karate or judo then what about tai chi or Qi Gong?

Or have a full body massage and let yourself go. Rather than checking your to do lists, use the time during the massage to pay close attention to what is happening in your body and how it affects you.

Laughter

Have a good old belly laugh. There doesn't need to be a reason.

I remember as a child that we would be sitting around the dinner table and my father would suddenly announce "Let's have a jolly good laugh!" He would lead the way, chuckling and laughing and before long we were all helpless with laughter, tears streaming down our faces.

I recently attended my first Laughter Yoga class and was struck by the similarity.

Throw caution to the wind and laugh like you used to in math class when you knew you were about to get in trouble for laughing. Feel that abandonment where you don't need to know why you are laughing, it is just happening anyway.

Clear out, clean up

Review your kitchen cupboard and see if there are some things you want to get rid of because you know intuitively that they are not what your body or digestion system is needing these days.

If you're not sure, try holding the thing in your hand and either use muscle testing if you are familiar with that, or just sense if it is empowering or disempowering for you. Restock with food options that feel right for you and use them regularly for a month to see if your habits shift.

Sound support

You can also hum or chant to attune this chakra. The Sanskrit sound for the sacral chakra is RAM (pronounced romm) and the note on the Western scale is E.

How: ...Solar plexus chakra

As for the other chakras, listening to music designed for this chakra as you go about your day will also help heal and balance it. Search the Sanskrit name on YouTube for lots of examples, maybe start to make your own playlist with your favorites for each chakra.

Nutritional support

Yellow foods help rebalance and strengthen the solar plexus chakra. Think of corn, yellow peppers, bananas, squash, pineapple, yellow lentils, chickpeas and amaranth - an ancient kind of grain that is gluten free and high in protein.

Recipe for Yellow Sunshine pie

Ingredients

Filling

- 2 corncobs
- a handful of pine nuts
- a drizzle of olive oil
- 1 onion, diced finely
- 1 yellow pepper, diced finely
- 1 cup sour cream
- 1 egg (optional)

Pastry

- 2 cups amaranth flour
- 4 tablespoons of coconut oil (the more natural the better)

How: …Solar plexus chakra

- ½ cup of water
- pinch of salt

Instructions

1. Preheat your oven to 200C/400F
2. Boil the corncobs for 5-10 minutes till they look juicy and ready to go.
3. While they are cooking, dry roast the pine kernels to bring out the flavor. Keep an eye on them because they burn very quickly. Keep them on the move. Remove from the frying pan.
4. Add a drizzle of olive oil to the pan and gently fry the onion and pepper until soft and starting to become golden brown.
5. Drain and shuck the corn (cut off the corn kernels) and discard the center of the corn cob. Blend with sour cream and an egg if you eat them, and season to taste. Use egg and cream substitute for a vegan alternative.
6. Put the mixture to one side while you make the pastry.
7. Put the flour in a blender and add the salt then the oil. Dribble in the water until the dough forms a ball.
8. Press the dough out into a circle on a greased baking sheet with a slightly thicker rim so it can contain the filling. Or use a flan dish or shallow pie dish. I like to bake it blind (cover with greaseproof paper and baking blind beans if you have them) for 10-15

minutes first so that it is crispier. Or you can go straight to the next step.

9. Cover the dough with the onion pepper mix and pour over the corn batter. Sprinkle the pine nuts on top.
10. Cook for 15-20 mins until firm and golden and serve with a tomato salad.

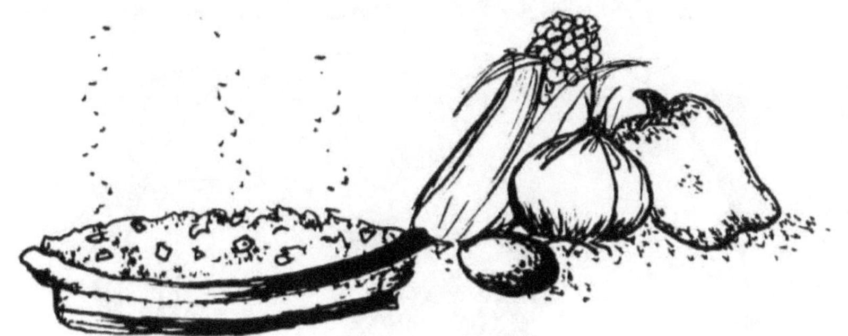

Heart chakra

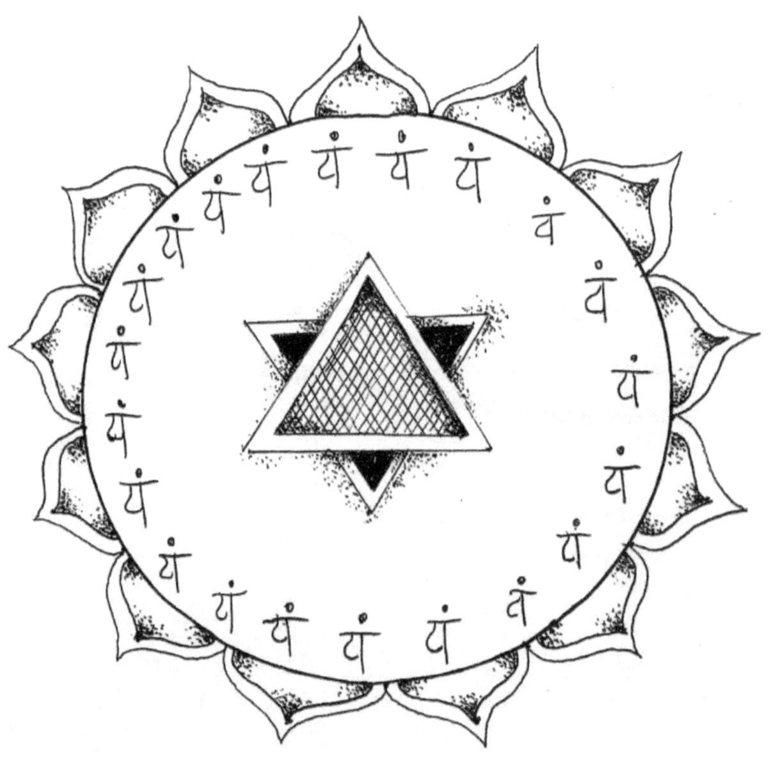

Information about the heart chakra

Introduction

Our heart chakra is located close to our physical heart, centrally in the body. Not surprisingly, it is associated with love.

That includes romantic love, but it primarily relates to universal love. The love we give and receive with other people, animals, places and situations. The compassion we feel when we hear the plight of a people or person struck by natural disaster or war. The sense of gratitude we feel when a complete stranger helps us out.

This chakra concept of love is the connection we all have with each other whenever we are open to it. Not a cautious love to be meted out in careful rations, according to merit and tallied on a mental reckoning sheet. But an infinite pool of unconditional love that we can give of freely. Indeed, it is many people's experience that the more love we give, the more there is available.

The best place to start is with yourself, since then you will benefit both from the giving of love and the receiving of it. This will help to build a deep well of love for you to share with others.

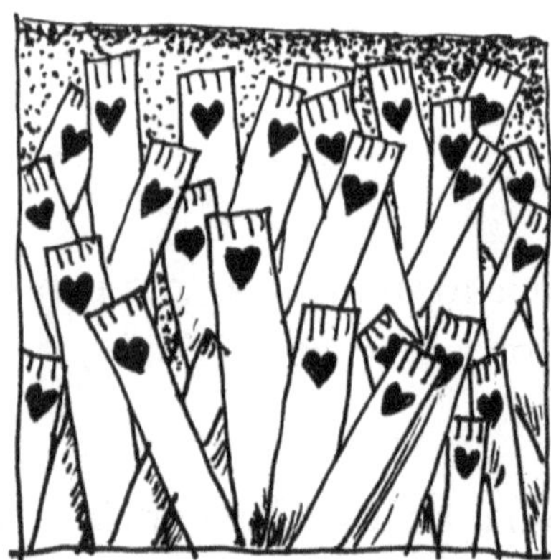

Can you look yourself in the eyes in a mirror for several minutes and then say, "I love you"? And mean it?

You might find it hard at first. You might experience feelings of shame, self-loathing – or just feel awkward. Give yourself the experience of trying it each time you look in the mirror for 21 days and see if anything shifts. Many people find this is an important first step for them to expand the experience and quantity of love in their life.

Giving love generates the same feel-good hormones in our body as receiving it – and is something we can more easily choose. Yet it has been seen as weakness in some circles. Of course, it suits the army general or the CEO or the cosmetics marketer for us to feel a lack of love. Who can easily love a man and then kill him? Or destroy someone else's business for the sake of our own.? Who can encourage spending by making someone feel ugly or fat or inadequate in some other way if they love them?

How: …Heart chakra

We have been trained out of giving love freely by a world where some actions are driven by fear and suspicion. And then we are offered consumer goods as a soother for the sense of loss. That new pair of trainers or the latest mobile phone may well give you some endorphins for a while. But you could get the same chemicals and feelings for free in other ways - that are more enduring.

Physically this chakra is associated of course with the heart, and also the lungs. These organs are closely related – the two things we check to establish life. Or preserve it in the case of CPR.

Our whole body relies on the transportation of oxygen as fuel to our cells – to work optimally this requires health and balance in both lungs and heart. The heart, like the gut, also has a significant cluster of nerve cells.

The heart is also the greatest center of electromagnetic energy in the body. Small wonder that we feel unaccountably drawn to some people. Their magnetic field is resonating with ours.

We all understand what it means to be heavy-hearted. And the liberating sense of a wave of light-heartedness. Bring light into your heart whenever you can. It does not make you superficial or trivial. Far from it. It is like oxygen in society, helping us through good times and bad.

As you go about your heart chakra focus day, experiment with holding and sharing more love. For the sheltering sky. For the refrigerator that preserves your food. For the farmer who produced it. For the train driver who transports you. For the person who sells you your morning newspaper or coffee. You don't need to tell them, just feel it in your heart chakra and they will sense it at some level.

Color

Although pink and red have become strongly associated with romantic love, the color of this chakra is actually green. Representing universal love. The color of abundance. In our primitive state, green indicated a possible food source or the first signs of spring. Both essential to our survival.

And because green is in the middle of the visible part of the electromagnetic spectrum (the rainbow), it is the easiest color for our eye to rest on.

I try always to work somewhere from which I can see green. Ideally natural but if that isn't possible, then a picture or piece of fabric is a good substitute. Or a pot plant! The sight of green calms the nervous system.

Turn up your color green to increase the love in your life – both giving and receiving.

Element

The heart chakra element is air. A spacious, clear, life force. Something we all have in common. The air that I breathe may have been breathed by you in the past. It connects us all with its life-giving blend of just the right amount of oxygen.

How: …Heart chakra

From our very first breath that signals the start of life to our last breath indicating we have moved on the average person will breathe two thirds of a billion times in their life. It is worth paying attention to a few of those breaths to nourish our well-being.

Prana, or breath, life force makes a huge difference to our well-being. It is the single most accessible tool we have at our disposal. Try breathing very fast and shallow, so only your chest or shoulders move. How does that make you feel? Your automatic systems assume there is an emergency eg running away from a tiger, so they start producing stress hormones and sending your blood away from your central organs and brain into your limbs. It makes sense, in that situation, to prioritize energy into running away than into digesting lunch.

The issue is that a lot of our stress in the modern world has very little to do with being chased by a tiger. It might be triggered by worrying about that meeting with your anger prone boss, looking at this month's bank statement or noticing a repeated and worrying behavior in your spouse or teenage child.

None of these situations are likely to require running at great speed. They are however likely to benefit from equanimity, calmness, quick thinking and good decision-making capacity. To trigger our physical system to be ready for this, we can use our prana, our breath, and make ourselves breathe slowly and deeply so only our belly moves.

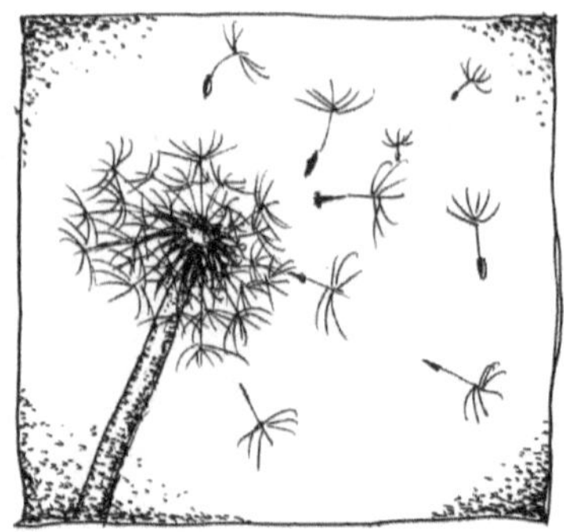

Without doing anything else, this change in breathing style will start to improve our coping capacity as the brain triggers a different cocktail of calming hormones.

Consider too the range of air movements in the world. From the gentlest whispering breeze to a mighty hurricane. Like fire, it is considered a masculine element (compared to earth or water, which is feminine). Air as wind powers sailing boats and wind turbines, transports seeds for germination and allowed us to expand our view of the earth from a few miles or kilometers to across oceans to other continents thanks to the so-called winds of discovery, or trade winds.

Name and Symbol

Anahata, the Sanskrit name for the heart chakra is made up of the words *ana* – un – and *hata* – hurt. What a beautiful concept of universal love. To love like a newborn child. As though we had never been let down or betrayed. To love freely and fearlessly. No trace of withholding.

How: …Heart chakra

This kind of unconditional love is not easy, but it is worth holding as an intention, even as we accept that we might never achieve it. Try the heart meditation later in this chapter to expand your love freedom.

In the symbol for this chakra we see the combination of the inverted triangle (feminine energy) and the upright triangle (masculine energy). Accepting both is part of our path to feeling more comfortable with ourselves.

We all need this unity. Our masculine energy gives us the drive to get things done, the structures that give shape to our days. While our feminine energy helps us connect with others and harness our creativity and intuition. Both are present in each of us, whether we present as male or female or non-binary. Both are of value and make a great team!

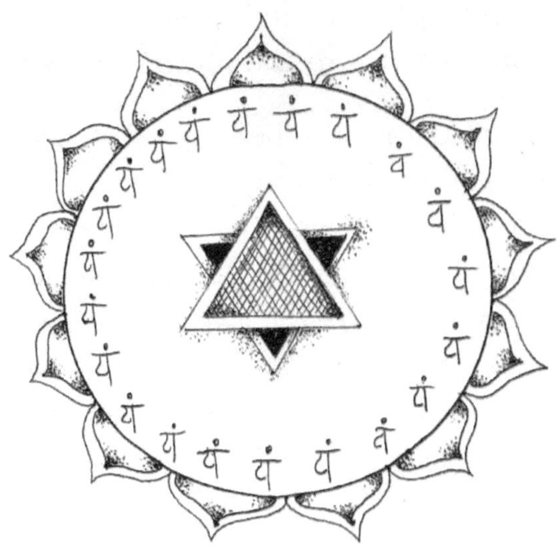

How: …Heart chakra

Honor both in yourself.

Around the circle are 12 petals representing 12 aspects that can help us on our path to love. These are peace, bliss, love, harmony, empathy, understanding, purity (of intent), clarity, compassion, unity, forgiveness and kindness. When you find it hard to feel love for someone or something in your life, maybe because of past hurt, you may be able to access love through sending them one of these other emotions instead.

Signs of imbalance in the heart chakra

Physical signs

An excess of energy in this chakra, or a blockage is associated with heart function issues such as arrhythmia, high or low blood pressure and in extremis, heart attacks.

As this chakra also governs the lungs, it is also connected with lung disease ranging from a wheezy cough to life threatening conditions. If you have ever experienced lung conditions that make you wheeze give you shortness of your breath, you may recognize the impulse to close in around your heart rather than open it. If you are aware of this tendency you can choose to respond differently and feed this chakra rather than starving it.

Emotional and psychological signs

A wounded or broken heart can have long term consequences. We can easily build up defenses around our heart. Like the thorn bushes that grew up around Sleeping Beauty's castle and kept everyone away. It might happen bit by bit – a series of small disappointments, knockbacks from people we care about or regrets from missed opportunities. Or it could be a sudden brutal blow like the loss of someone close to us, creating a pain we feel we can scarcely survive.

These things can happen in the course of a life. And while I wouldn't wish to diminish these events in any way whatsoever, it may be that nurturing your heart chakra can help your healing process.

Allowing your heart to gradually open to love again. Cutting down some of those thorn bushes yourself.

Or you could wait patiently for Prince Charming to make his way through, but rumor has it that takes 100 years and you might find that a bit too long to wait!

Also associated with low energy in this chakra is a struggle to love or accept yourself. Maybe the negative voices in your head have the upper hand and you feel yourself to be unlovable.

The good news is you can heal this. Try the heart meditation below (or listen to it on my you tube channel Winds of Discovery). Try EFT (see video on my channel for that too) or any other practice where you gradually shift your feelings about yourself. It took me many years to be able to say "I love myself" so don't be disheartened if this is the case for you too. Just keep working on it and you will get there. From personal experience I can say it is well worth the effort. Once you love yourself, loving anybody else is easier.

Supporting your heart chakra

Yoga support

(See supporting video on youtube.com/catherineshovlin)

Our yoga postures for this chakra will have an aspect of softness. This is definitely not about pushing yourself to extremes. Move gently and slowly, as though you were trying not to disturb the air around you at all.

Heart warming

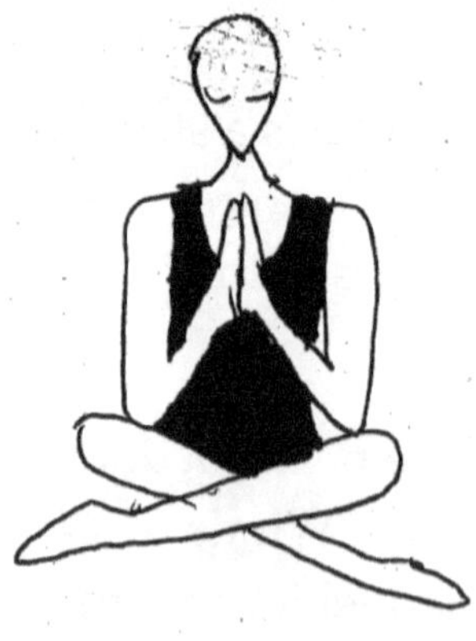

How: …Heart chakra

Take a comfortable seat on the mat in easy pose (cross
legged). Or sit in a chair or on a cushion if that is more
comfortable for you.

Bring your hands together into prayer position and rest your
thumbs against your heart. Breathe softly through your nose
for 5 breaths and be aware of the gentle soothing pressure on
your heart.

When we feel this gentle pressure here against our sternum,
we release endorphins – nature's way of encouraging us to
carry babies around.

Airy heart

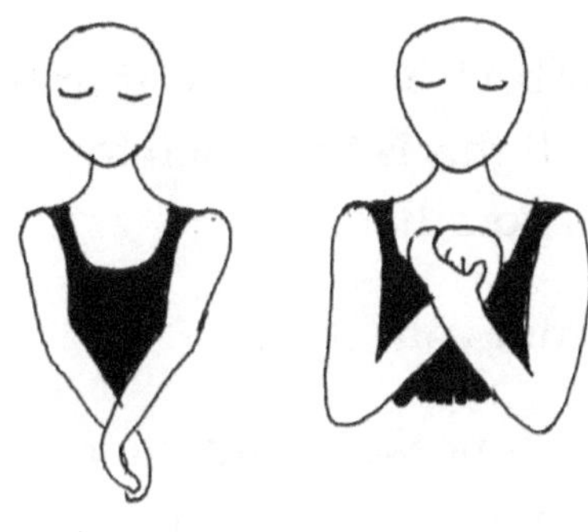

Stretch your arms out in front of you and cross your right
arm over the left at the wrists.

Turn your palms to face each other and clasp your hands.

Spread your elbows as you rotate your still clasped hands
down and back up, so they are turned over and your clasped
knuckles are close to your body. Rest your clasped hands
against your heart chakra and take 5 slow, deep breaths.

How: …Heart chakra

Release your hands and shake out your wrists if necessary.Repeat starting with the left arm crossed over the right.

Heart opening

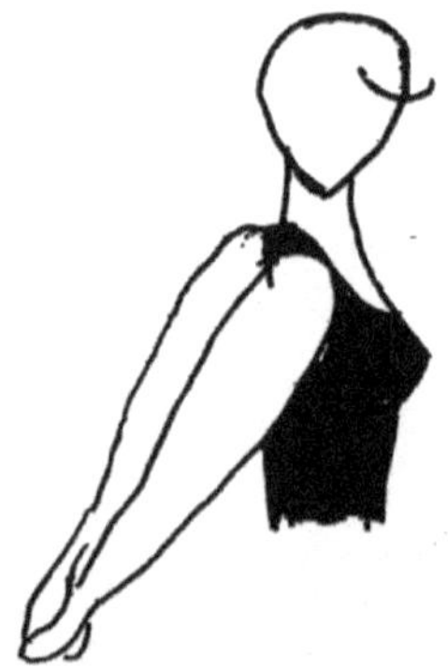

Next clasp your hands behind your back and pull your arms straight and away from your body. If this is too much for you, hold the opposite elbows with your hands.

Now lift your arms up and away from your back.

This is a good counterpose to all the time we spend hunched over a keyboard, sewing machine, mobile phone, baby, steering wheel….

Feel your shoulder blades tucking in towards each other and your collar bones and heart area opening up. Inhale and really enjoy the stretch and creation of space around your lungs and heart.

Exhale and lower your hands towards your back. Inhale and raise them, exhale and lower. Do that 5 times in total.

Airy ribcage

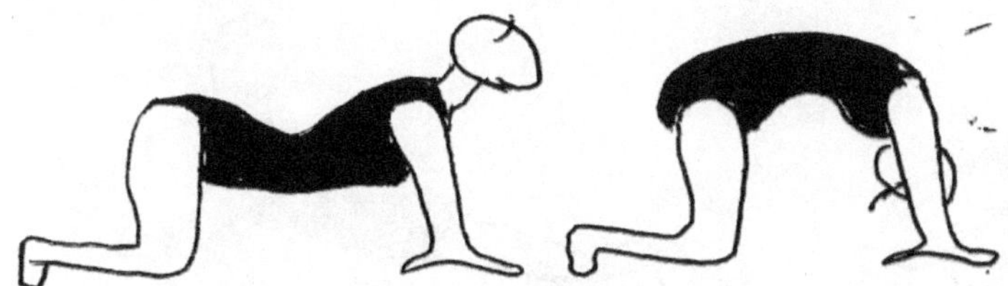

Place your hands on the mat in front of you and come up onto all fours. We will do a few rounds of cat-cow pose here, gently and playfully.

See if you can have a smile on your face as you inhale, arching your back and raising your chin, then exhale as you curve your back upwards, and drop your head, chin towards chest.

Do 5 repetitions like this and then try playing with the posture.

What would feel good for your body right now? Maybe moving your hips or shoulders left and right. Maybe swirling your hips in a circle. Feel into what are the juiciest poses for you and let yourself enjoy them. Your body knows best what it needs.

Airy breastbone

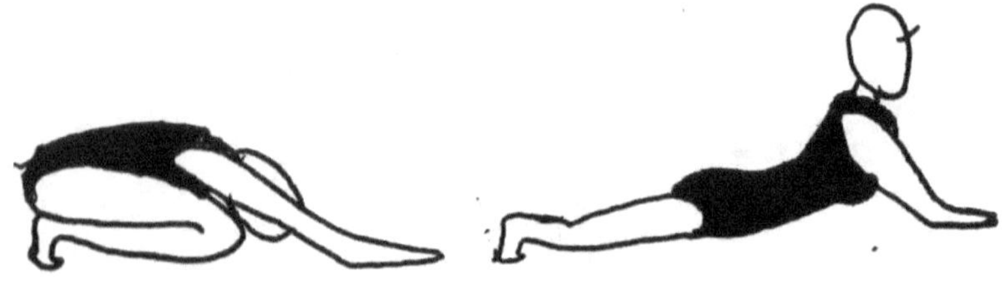

Keeping your hands on the ground, exhale as you move your hips back and down onto your heels in child's pose.

Inhale and come forward onto your elbows in sphinx pose. Lift your sternum forward and up. Feel your heart opening.

Exhale and flow back into child's pose, then inhale forward into sphinx.

Keep this flowing movement going for a few more rounds and notice how it makes your heart chakra feel warmer and more open.

Lionheart

Now sit back on your heels for lion pose. Heels together, knees apart. Settle into the ground and feel strong. Rest your hands on your knees.

How: …Heart chakra

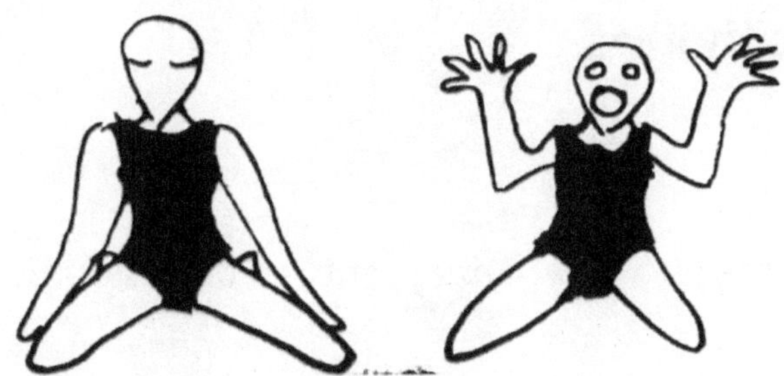

Take a deep inhale and then as you exhale raise your hands
to the sides of your face, palms facing forwards, fingers
spread as wide as you can.

Stretch your eyes wide open as well as your mouth. (Yes,
you will look a bit mad… that's part of the fun!)

Let your breath out with a hah! sound – or even a roar if that
feels right for you.

Repeat 5 times.

Advanced

For more experienced yoga practitioners, camel, wheel or
bridge pose are also good for opening the heart chakra.

Supporting activities

Self-love

Practice the art of self-love. There are plenty of books on this topic.

To start with just place your hands on your sternum (breastbone) and gently breathe in and out. Imagine you are breathing through your heart. Close your eyes.

You might do this lying down to be even more relaxed. Put cushions under your elbows and knees for more support and an even greater sense of being held. Stay like that for at least five minutes without moving, to allow the endorphins to kick in.

Once you are used to accessing the feeling you can do it with just one hand on your heart at any time when you feel the need for a bit more support. This is something we do almost unconsciously, we are just raising the awareness a little to increase the benefit.

Check your breathing signature

Are you breathing shallowly? Just using the top part of your lungs?

To find out your breathing signature, lie on the floor on your back and place one hand on your belly and one on your chest. Just breathe naturally, in the way you usually do, and see how your body moves with your breath. Do you breathe more in your belly or in your chest?

Breathing lower in your body involves your diaphragm. It is this moving downwards that causes your belly to swell rather than air going into your belly as of course your lungs are in your chest cavity.

If that horizontal sheet of muscle known as the diaphragm has weakened from lack of use, or disease, then you may find you are breathing primarily in the upper part of your lungs, moving your chest. You may also be doing this habitually without any physical reason.

Changing the way in which you breathe can have a fundamental effect on your well-being. Some yogis say it can add ten years to your life.

To check this out for yourself, deliberately breathe using just the top of your lungs for ten breaths. You will need to breathe more frequently as you can take in less air this way. What do you notice? What feelings do you have? Maybe a vague sense of anxiety, or being under pressure? Of instability?

Then switch to belly breathing. Try not to move your chest or shoulders at all but feel the air expanding the lower part of your lungs, pushing the diaphragm down and the belly out. Do this for ten breaths and then again observe how you are feeling.

How: …Heart chakra

Remember the difference this makes in the hormones secreted by your system, as described in the introduction.

Moments of stress and anxiety may well be some of the hardest times to make ourselves breathe differently. But if you can find the presence and self-love to do so then you will feel the benefit.

Healing love

Think of your earliest memory of feeling that you were not loved. Or not loved in the way that you needed to be.

Maybe you were a small child, or even a baby. And something somebody said or did triggered the fear of abandonment. At that age we need other people in order to survive, so the fear of them not loving us is primal and strong. It could mean a matter of life and death.

Imagine you are there now, as your adult self. Pick up this young version of yourself and give him or her a big hug. Shower them with love. Ask them how they feel and acknowledge their feelings. You don't need to fix anything or explain anything. Just allow them to share how they feel and accept that they feel that way.

Then tell them how much you love them and that you will always be there for them, no matter what. Tell them that as many times as it takes to sink into their heart.

Get your heart pumping!

Get some cardiovascular exercise. No need to bust a gut, a brisk walk or a few runs up and down the stairs will do it. Find something you enjoy doing that gets your heart energized. See if you can do ten minutes a day and then gradually increase it. Know your limits, listen to your body, build up gradually.

As my homeopath always tells me, a stout heart is a very useful thing to have.

Share love

I find this one helpful on a train, in doctor's waiting room or any other situation where I might feel a bit uncomfortable or just bored, and there are other people in the space not interacting much with each other.

Look at each person in turn (discreetly!). Imagine they have just shared something that is on their mind. A problem with a pet or a lover or a family member. Maybe an issue at work or something social. Reassure them. Tell them it's going to be ok. That you are on their side and you believe in them. (All of this is in your head of course, not out loud unless you are very confident!).

Move on to the next person. As you work your way around the room or train carriage you might start to feel the atmosphere shift.

How: ...Heart chakra

You have raised the love vibration of the space. That's good
for all the people you have sent love to – and it's good for
you too. You might get a kick out of this compassionate
intervention and the fact that nobody will ever know it was
you.

Sing your heart out

Singing is a great way to open your heart. It doesn't matter
whether you think you "can sing" - so many of us are told
we cannot when we are growing up and this can shut us
down. Now is the time to put that aside and sing anyway.

Singing also connects to the next chakra, the throat. The
heart and throat chakra have a very close relationship.

Find something you love that you can sing along to, or just
make random sounds. It doesn't matter. You might find you
don't even recognize the voice that comes through you. That
also doesn't matter. Let it soar. The words don't need to
make sense, or even be recognizable in any language you are
familiar with. The most important thing is to let it out.

The shower is the traditional place for this – you may also
find it easier to sing when you are driving a car alone with
the radio on full blast, playing with children or in a remote
landscape a long way from anybody who might overhear.

Practice gratitude

300 years before positive psychology developed, Émilie du
Châtelet, accomplished mathematician also famous for being

How: …Heart chakra

Voltaire's mistress, kept a happiness journal to help her cope with the ups and downs of life as an unacknowledged female scientist (she had to publish her translation of Newton's works under a man's name) and supporter / comforter of a controversial and outspoken character like Voltaire.

Each day she would write 3 things that she appreciated about the day. A gratitude diary.

This is a fascinating habit to take up. I had no idea I got satisfaction from cleaning up the kitchen until I started this! I also realized how the things we might do in pursuit of happiness - like having a glass of wine, opening a bar of chocolate or going shopping – tend not to show up in the list.

It is interesting to observe your own patterns so that you can start to shift your life towards the things that make you feel good. Things you love. And also to help you realize that even on a bad day there were some bright spots.

Sound support

As well as singing, you can also hum or chant to attune this chakra. The Sanskrit sound for the heart chakra is YAM (pronounced yomm) and the note in the Western musical scale is F.

Make yourself a Love Playlist. You might want to include some romantic songs, and also think about those that speak of a more universal love - of brother/sisterhood, compassion or solidarity. Songs like Stand by me, Venceremos or What the world needs now…

Play your Love Playlist for yourself whenever you want to reconnect with other people. Or for others when you want to subtly bring more love into the space.

Nutritional support

You won't be surprised to hear that getting your greens is good for your heart. Any green vegetables will help, and also other green things like spirulina or matcha / green tea.

If you're not keen on eating them then get the blender out and chuck them in there. Add some green apples for sweetness, limes for sharpness or avocado for creaminess according to your preferences. Include coconut water or apple juice to get the consistency the way you want it, and ice if you like a smoother texture. It's easy to add a teaspoonful of green spirulina powder to increase the nutrients.

For the more sweet-toothed of you, try this recipe to warm your heart.

How: …Heart chakra

Recipe for Love Cookies

Ingredients

- 2 tbsp butter or alternative
- 1 tbsp honey, maple syrup or another natural sweetener
- 1 cup almond flour or equivalent
- 1 cup of cold black or green tea (without milk)
- 2 cups of your favorite dried fruits. You can add candied fruit too if you like
- 1 cup of chopped nuts (optional)
- 1 cup of granola
- A pinch or two of cinnamon, mixed spice or cardamom seeds (not the pods) according to what takes your fancy

Instructions

This is an easy one.

1. Preheat the oven to 180 C / 350 F
2. Melt the butter or margarine and stir in the syrup or honey.
3. Stir in the flour and cook for a minute, stirring all the time.
4. Gradually add the tea, stirring to avoid lumps.
5. Heat until just beginning to boil then turn off the heat
6. Stir in all the other ingredients.
7. If you need to adjust the consistency, add more flour or tea.

8. Press into a greased baking tray and cook for 15 mins.

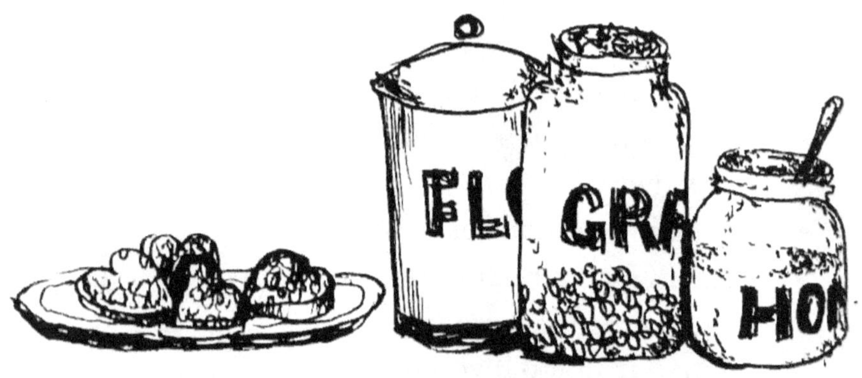

Throat chakra

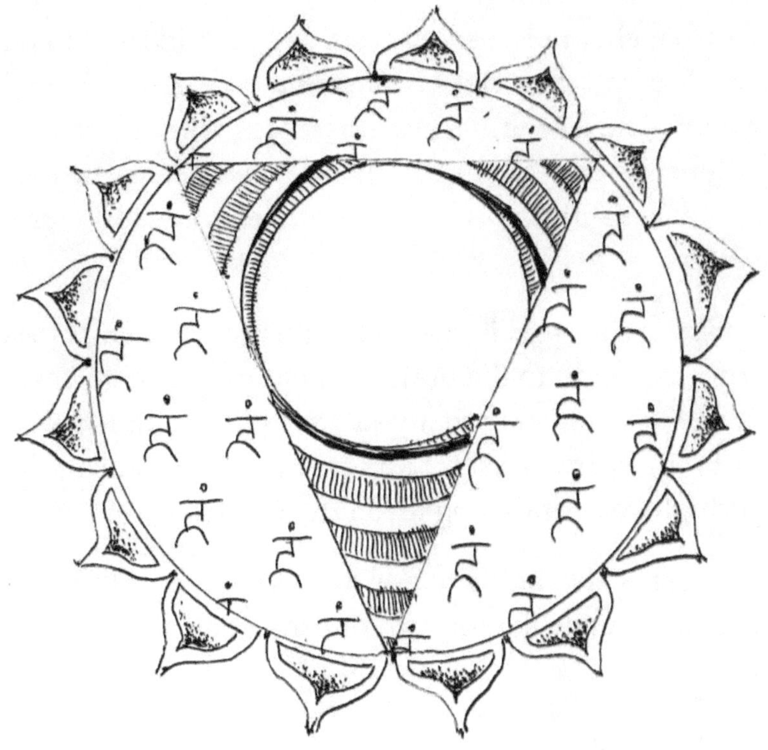

Information about the throat chakra

Introduction

The throat chakra is, as you would expect, located in our throat. That all important connection between our mind and our body. Under normal circumstances, through this "bottleneck" pass all the air that we breathe, all the food and drink that sustains us and every sound, song and word that we utter.

Our nervous system is channeled this way too on its way to or from the body to the brain. Every time your skin sends a message to your brain that you are feeling a bit too warm, or your brain instructs your hand to move, the message superhighway is hurtling through your throat chakra.

The throat is also home to our thyroid and parathyroid – important organs that govern our metabolism and bone health.

With all this going on, it is no surprise that this chakra governs communication. Both internally – is your brain listening to your heart? Is your heart listening to your brain? – and externally – are you speaking your truth? Being heard? Having your say?

Color

The color of this chakra is a clear aqua blue. The color on the horizon where the sea meets a cloudless sky.

How: …Throat chakra

My bathroom is tiled in this color and I notice that some people describe it as blue – leaning more towards the next chakra, the third eye governing the brain. While others describe it as green – the color of the heart chakra.

I am always intrigued by this and indeed I now see that the more heart centered people are more likely to say green while the more intellectual say blue.

Great communication is a balance of the two. Using the clarity and observation of the brain alongside the compassion and good intention of the heart. You do not have to choose if you let your heart rule your head or vice versa. You can help them operate as a team.

Physiologically, the color blue stimulates brainwave activity. This lighter end of the spectrum is a more open and outward facing kind of intellect. More about our intellectual relationship with the world and less about the pure intellectual activities we might pursue in our inner world. This unique position midway between the body and the mind can be a beautiful combination of love and knowledge – or a conflict zone.

Tune into the beautiful possibilities of this color and sing out your truth.

Element

The element associated with the throat chakra – and all of these three higher chakras (throat, third eye, crown) is ether. The spaciousness in the universe.

Ether is also described as the carrier of sound – very relevant for a chakra that is all about communication and having a voice.

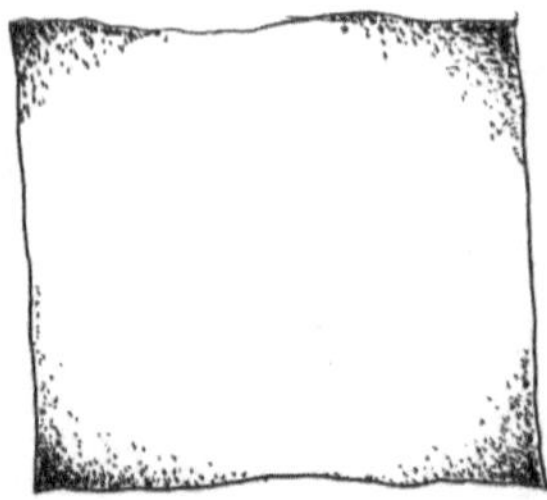

It is said that while the other four ancient elements (earth, air, fire and water) move in straight lines, ether moves in circles. Linear time and space are not a constraint. The alchemists refer to it as quintessence – that elusive quality that could be the elixir of life, the cure to everything. The term has been revived by some scientists trying to understand the mysteries of the dark energy that makes up two thirds of the universe and is thought to drive its accelerating expansion.

All that we have ever seen or measured or detected on earth and in space adds up to about 5% of the universe. The rest is dark energy or dark matter. Ether contains a lot to discover and we are just at the beginning of that journey as Albert Einstein realized last century that space is not 'empty'

Name and Symbol

The throat chakra's Sanskrit name *Vishuddha,* means "very pure". It has a 16 petalled lotus flower as its symbol. In the center is the inverted triangle and circle that is the seed element for ether.

The 16 petals are said to be associated with the vowel sounds in Sanskrit. In any language, the vowels create the airiness in words, the formed space between the consonants that allows us to understand. This interpretation makes sense for the communication aspect of the throat chakra.

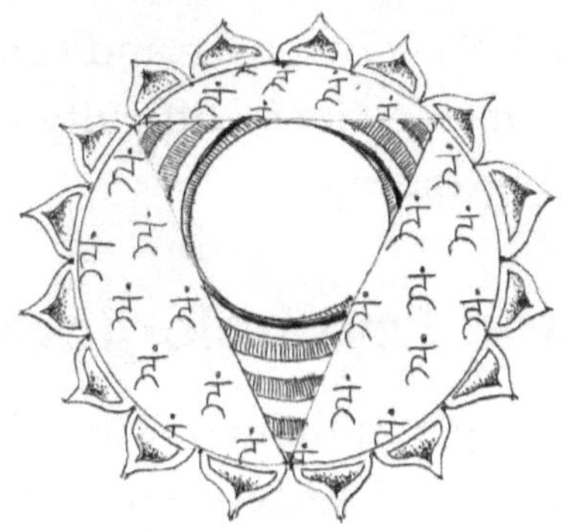

Signs of imbalance in the throat chakra

Physical signs

These days our throat chakra has more pressure and less exercise than has been the case for our ancestors so it may be prone to blockages.

If you spend a lot of time with your head bowed towards a screen, you may feel the effects in the short term with a stiff neck or shoulders as well as sore throats. Longer term this can affect your voice or thyroid function – hypoactive or hyperactive depending on whether you throat chakra is low energy or blocked.

This chakra is also associated with hearing and jaw problems. (Think ENT – Ear, nose and throat specialists) such as tinnitus, ear infections, difficulty swallowing, toothache or teeth grinding.

Emotional and Psychological signs

We talk about having a lump in our throat when we are upset. We also talk about someone or something having a stranglehold – just to hear that word triggers a primal reaction in us. And we may find a situation "hard to swallow".

If you feel that you are not speaking up for yourself, suffering from shyness that stops you living the life you want to live, not speaking your truth or feeling choked up you may want to rebalance your throat chakra energy. Connect your head to your heart and tackle any lack of integrity between how you present yourself to the world and who you really are.

If you work in the creative field and find yourself suffering from writer's block – or its equivalent in your area, it might be worth spending some time on your throat chakra to free up your creativity again.

Those with issues around their throat chakra may also have difficulty knowing what they really want – or asking for it.

Supporting your throat chakra

Yoga support

(See supporting video on youtube.com/catherineshovlin)

We can use yoga to open and stretch out our throat to help the energy flow more freely between our head and our body - and bring spaciousness into our being.

Throat awareness

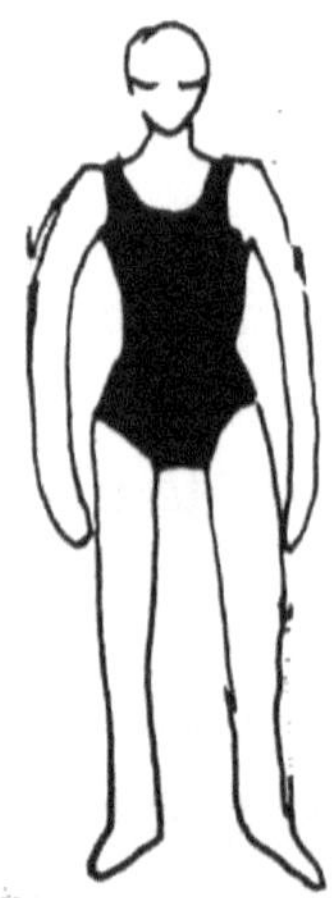

Start in a standing position, feet hip-width apart and arms relaxed by your sides (mountain pose).

Settle your weight so that it is spread evenly between left and right foot, as well as the front and back of the foot.

Pull up your kneecaps softly and straighten your pelvis.

Allow your shoulders to move away from your ears as your shoulder blades pull gently towards your spine.

Check your chin is level with the floor. Relax your jaws and around your eyes.

Throughout the following movements, practice ocean (*ujjayi*) breath. If this is new to you, the technique is to breathe through your nose, mouth closed. Slightly constrict the back of your throat as though you were going to whisper. You will hear the breathy sound of the air moving in and out.

How: …Throat chakra

The sound of this breath is often likened to the sound of waves ebbing and flowing on the seashore. This is especially noticeable when you have a roomful of people all using this breath.

Throat Opening

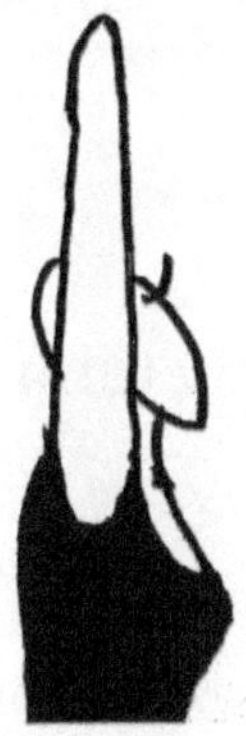

Still in the same standing position, inhale with ocean breath as you raise your arms up to the sky and lift your head up and slightly back to open the front of your throat.

Exhale towards the sky with an "aah!" sound.

Inhale as you bring your hands together above your head, palm to palm, and straighten your head. Exhale as you lower your hands down, palms still together, past your third eye, nose, lips, throat and heart.

Relax your arms back by your sides and repeat the whole cycle 5 times in total.

Baby neck

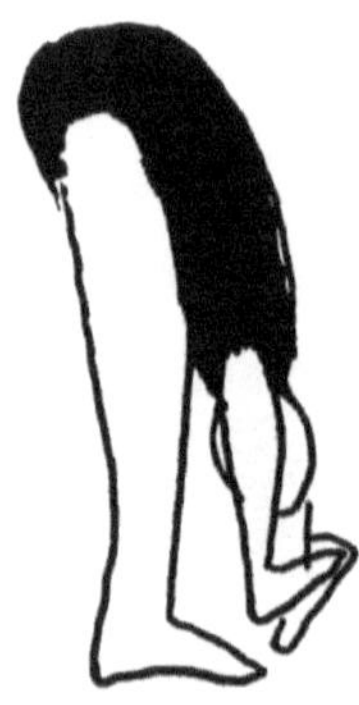

Now still standing, inhale and lift your rib cage away from your hips, raising your arms up to the sky.

Exhale as you slowly bend from the hips into a forward bend. Go to the place that feels like a comfortable stretch for you. It is fine to bend your knees; this is not about stretching your hamstrings.

Take hold of opposite elbows with your hands and let your head dangle down. If you have ever held a very young baby, you will know how they don't yet have the neck strength to support their heads. Imagine that wobbly, free baby neck and let your head jiggle around a bit.

Enjoy the sensation of the vertebrae at the back of your neck releasing tension.

Neck stretch

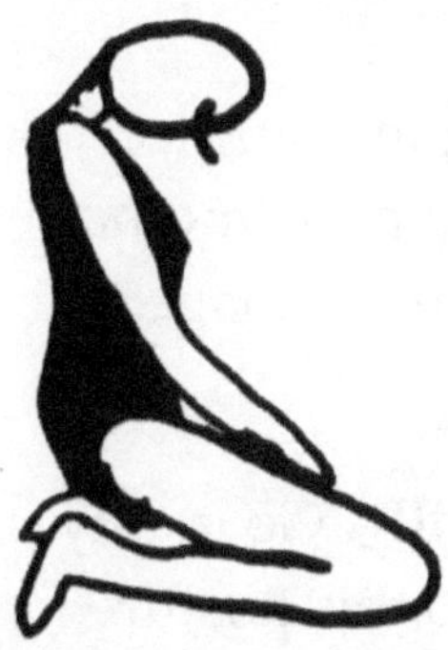

Staying in a forward bend, put your hands on the ground (bend your knees if you need to) and then lower yourself to sit down on your heels. Use a cushion between your bottom and your heels if that makes you more comfortable. Or if you have trouble with your knees find another seated position that works for you.

Now we are going to rotate our necks. Before we start, make sure your shoulders are relaxed, shoulder blades drawn down your back and gently towards each other, back straight, jaw relaxed.

Inhale and then as you exhale drop your head forward towards your chest. Don't try to push it down, just let it fall down. Notice where you are holding on, where there is resistance. Let that go. Relax into the posture, unclench your jaw, smooth away any frown-lines on your forehead.

Inhale as you roll your head round to the right, as though you were going to rest your right ear on your right shoulder.

How: …Throat chakra

Make sure your shoulder stays relaxed, resist the urge to raise it to meet your ear.

You may hear some clicking and crunching in your neck. So long as you are moving at your own natural pace and not pushing it, then you won't cause yourself any damage. Listen to your body and what it needs.

Exhale and roll your head to lean back slightly. Go gently on this back-leaning roll unless you are used to this posture.

Inhale and roll to the left as though you were putting your left ear on your left shoulder. Then exhale and roll around to the forward position, with your chin on, or moving towards, your chest.

Do this 4 times in this direction and then 4 times in the opposite direction.

Move slowly and gently, using the breath to help you while paying close attention to your body and what it is telling you.

Accept the clicks and 'coin chink' noises. Accept that one direction is easier than the other and one side of your neck more flexible than the other.

Imagine what it might be like to do this more regularly.

Strong neck

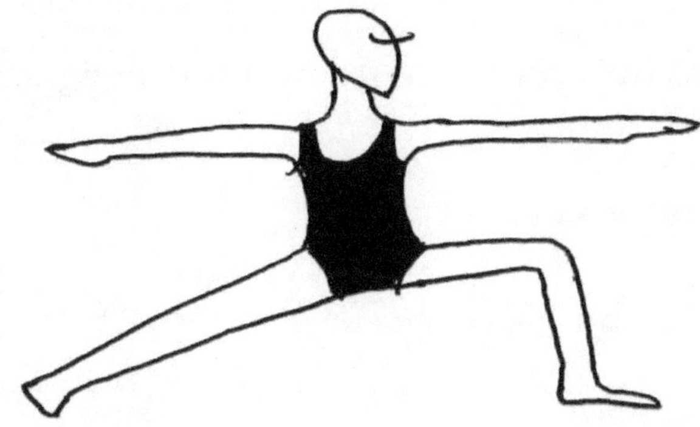

We will use Warrior 2 to bring our awareness to the strength of our neck.

Take a wide stance, (1.20-1.4m or 3.5-4 feet apart) and feel your power coming up from the earth through your feet.

Inhale and raise both arms to shoulder height, outstretched and with palms facing downwards.

Turn your left foot out to face the front of the mat and exhale as you bend your left leg, aiming for a right angle at the knee so your thigh is parallel to the floor and your shin is vertical.

Turn your head to look at your left hand.

Check your stance. Put as much weight into the ground on your back (right) foot as you do on the front one. Check your torso is upright, not leaning forward or twisting.

Stretch your arms wide without hunching your shoulders.

How: ...Throat chakra

Breathe deeply into your belly and imagine you are a glorious warrior, wise and strong.

After 5 deep breaths turn your head forward and straighten your left leg.

Now repeat to the other side.

Supporting activities

Singing or chanting

Of course, singing or chanting can be good for your throat chakra. But take care to approach it in the right way.

So many of us are self-conscious about our voices – maybe we were told once as children that we couldn't sing and have scarcely tried since then. I remember that whenever my sister and I used to sing our hearts out in church the people in the row in front would turn around and then turn back and look at each other and laugh. I have no idea what they were thinking but we both assumed the worst!

If you feel your throat constricting at the very idea of singing out loud, then make sure you have some privacy so you can relax. Maybe start with humming or lalala-ing.

For some people, imagining they are singing a lullaby to help baby get to sleep makes it easier. Others start with

How: …Throat chakra

something easy that they remember like a nursery rhyme or popular song, or a mantra or chant they are familiar with.

This is not about getting the notes or the tune or the words right. It is not about performing or perfecting.

It is about letting your throat do what it yearns for. To loosen and open and let the sound out. Maybe it's a murmur, maybe it's a roar.

Try to release any attachment to the outcome and just see what happens. Challenge yourself to making sounds for a full minute. Then work up to five minutes.

Sing or shout, laugh or cry - or do all of those.

If you are a confident singer, then give yourself the freedom to sing truly, madly, badly. Give up the idea of 'nice singing'.

When I did a workshop with the wonderful Chloe Goodchild (see her website thenakedvoice.com for more information) a few years ago, I startled myself with the sounds that came out of my mouth.

By the end of the day, the defining phrase that emerged for me was "my wild voice sings to my power". I have carried that with me ever since and it often brings me back to my truth as well as helping me sing or speak up.

Truth telling

Write a letter to yourself. The subject of the letter is "If only they knew".

In the letter, speak freely of all the things you keep hidden away. The things you only pretend to enjoy, the emotions that you do not feel comfortable expressing, the secret desires and hopes and fears. The shame, the regrets, the pride, the hidden talents, the secret crushes, the guilty secret habits.

Let it all come out, comfortable in the knowledge that nobody else is ever going to read it.

Keep going. Aim to write at least 2 or 3 pages. Writing by hand will have more impact than typing it on a keyboard. You may surprise yourself once you get into the flow and past the first, most obvious things.

Then find a space, ideally in nature a long way from anybody who might overhear and read the letter out loud. To the universe. By speaking your truth as you have written it, you are increasing your alignment with it.

You may find both the reading and the speaking aloud deeply uncomfortable, even painful. Particularly when you speak the words out loud, you might find strong emotions welling up. Relax your throat, let truth be told. Know that you will not be punished or mocked. Nobody is listening except the compassionate universe.

How: ...Throat chakra

Know too that everybody on the planet could write such a
letter and squirm at their truths. Or feel uncomfortable about
acknowledging their strengths. It is human.

Repeat this practice every day for a week. You might want to
use the same letter each day, or you might find it evolves
and goes deeper during the course of the week.

At the end of the week review your truths.

Are you getting any closer to saying some of them out loud
to the people who need to hear them? Consider that
possibility, and maybe find the safest person to start the
process. You could invite them to do the same, be truth
buddies for each other, with the understanding of total
confidentiality and safety.

When the other person reads out their letter, just listen with
your full attention. Don't react or comment or argue the
point. Listen like the sky. And thank them for sharing. That's
all. No observations, sympathy, discussion or 'helpful'
suggestions required. Ask them to do the same for you.

Sound support

The Sanskrit sound for the sacral chakra is HAM
(pronounced homm) and the note in the Western scale is G.

On YouTube you can find music that relates to this chakra
that you may enjoy listening to on the days when this is your
focus.

Nutritional support

The foods that support this area are exactly what you might associate with cough lozenges or medicine for sore throats. Soothing ingredients such as honey, lemon, coconut water and elderflower or elderberry-based drinks.

Another good source of support for this chakra are herbal teas, especially those containing licorice, sage, thyme or raspberry leaf (though this last one is best avoided during pregnancy).

Orchard fruits such as apples and pears also work well as do blue foods – though those are not common - moldy food is obviously not an option). Try blueberries, blackberries and purple cabbage or broccoli.

Recipe for throat soothing tea

You should be able to source all of these ingredients from your local health food shop or a good supermarket. I have suggested a blend here, but you might find you want a little more of something or less of something else. That's the beauty of making your own herbal tea, you can experiment until you find the blend that is exactly what you want.

How: …Throat chakra

Ingredients

- Licorice root
- Herbs: Rosemary, thyme, sage, borage (fresh or dried)
- Fruits: Blueberries, blackberries, leaves from blackberry or raspberry bushes. Can be fresh, frozen or dried.

Instructions

1. Let your instincts guide you and keep a note of what you add to your teapot so you can adjust if necessary next time.
2. Pour over freshly boiled water and leave for 5 minutes to allow the flavors to steep. If you like to drink your tea hot, cover the teapot with a tea-cozy (do people still have those? Maybe just me…) or just use a towel, woolly hat or scarf.
3. The way you drink the tea is as important as how you make it. Create a sacred moment for yourself. Get out your favorite cup, or the one you hardly ever use because you're saving it for a special moment. That moment is here now.
4. I like to use a teacup rather than a mug, when I have tea in a pot. As my grandmother explained to me, teacups are wider at the top than the bottom so the tea cools down fastest when the cup is full and slower as you go down as there is less surface area. That makes it the right temperature for more of the time.
5. Find a lovely place to sit. Maybe looking out over a favorite tree, or in a cozy armchair. Turn off your

phone, put down your work. Give yourself five minutes of precious restoration time.

6. Add honey if you want to. Notice the soothing attention of the tea moving down your throat, feeling it relaxing and opening. Know that you have a voice and can speak your truth.

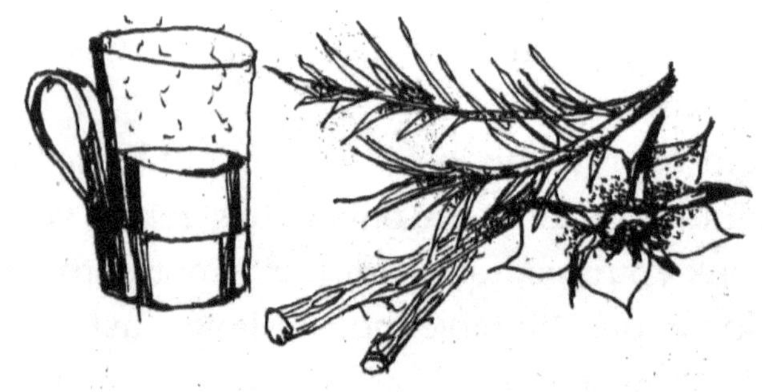

Third eye chakra

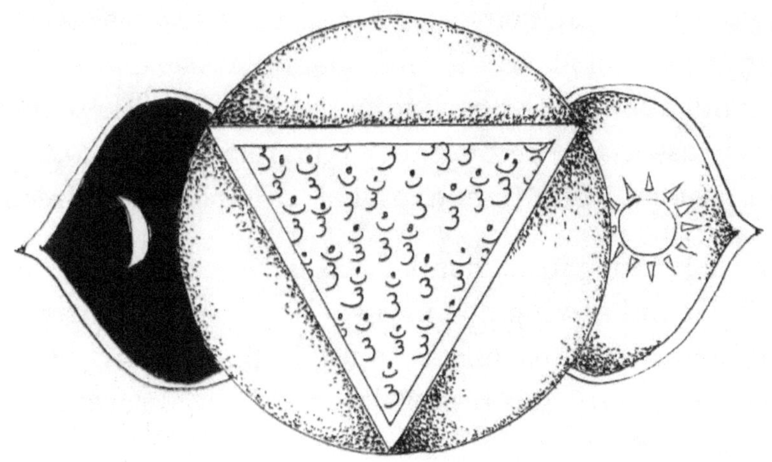

Information about the third eye chakra

Introduction

The Third Eye chakra, sometimes called the brow chakra is on your forehead, between your eyebrows and is associated with the pineal gland – a small gland the size and shape of a pine nut a few inches back from the third eye. These two are closely associated because they both relate to our connection with visions, visualization, psychic capability and dreams.

The role of the pineal gland – for many years thought to be vestigial and serving no purpose – is to produce melatonin – that in turn governs our circadian rhythm and triggers the onset of puberty. It is responsible for sleep patterns and sexual function.

This chakra is also associated with the pituitary gland, governing our endocrine system, and neighboring body parts – eyes, nose, ears, brain.

The pineal gland supports our ability to cope with change in an unpredictable world. It is believed to produce DMT, a similar substance to that found in drugs such as ayahuasca, used to access spiritual experiences, because it is instrumental in seeing visions, telepathy and lucid dreaming.

Even if your belief system does not accept these concepts, this chakra performs an important role in your discernment

– your bullshit detector to put it more prosaically, or your inbuilt GPS that helps you navigate through the world!

Some call it their Inner Guru – the source of our individual and collective wisdom and intuition. You may notice that when you are asked a question that you have to consider before answering, your eyes tend to look up and away from the person asking you, as though you might "see" the answer there.

A healthy third eye chakra will allow you to see the world and your role in it clearly. You will find it easier to visualize the path ahead and the actions that will support your future.

In kundalini yoga, many postures require the eyes to be focused on the third eye – inward and upward – to access this extension of ourselves and to see the Big Picture – the world or universe of which we are a part, not just considering everything from our own point of view.

Color

The color indigo (a dark purplish blue like the night sky) resonates with the Third Eye chakra. This is the color that stimulates intellectual activity, and indeed the third eye chakra is associated with brain activity.

In some cultures, meditating in the dark is used as a way to awaken the third eye and increase capacity to see visions. It is a form of seeing that does not require light.

How: …Third eye chakra

Imagine the feeling you get when you feel safe and can settle your gaze on the night sky. The hugeness of it. The possibilities, the scale, the comfort of feeling part of a bigger universe. Tune into the color indigo to find your depth and connection to the cosmos.

Element

As is the case for all three of the upper chakras, the element for the third eye chakra is ether. In this regard you might think of it as the space that allows us to see beyond everyday reality. To see auras or energy fields. To see emotions and connections between people in the room. To see ethereal bodies.

The act of seeing visions requires an emptying out of the mind, a ceasing of the mental chatter we engage in for much of the day and a falling into the silence beyond.

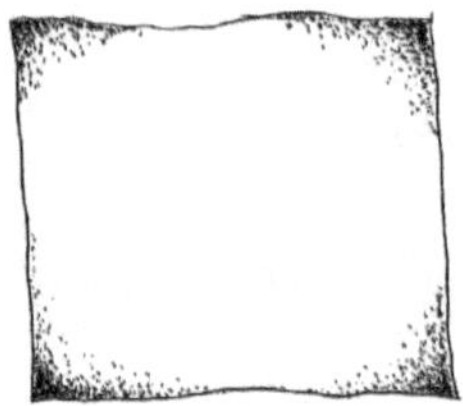

Name and Symbol

The Sanskrit name for this chakra is *Ajna*, meaning to *perceive* and to *command*. It also means spiritual connection. It is the highest chakra within our physical body so is given this name as it is the commander of our lower chakras – you may prefer to think of it as the conductor, like in an orchestra. It has a crucial two-way role of both perceiving what is happening in the environment (both those things that we can see or hear in the normal way and those happening at a higher vibration) and then organizing a response via the other chakras.

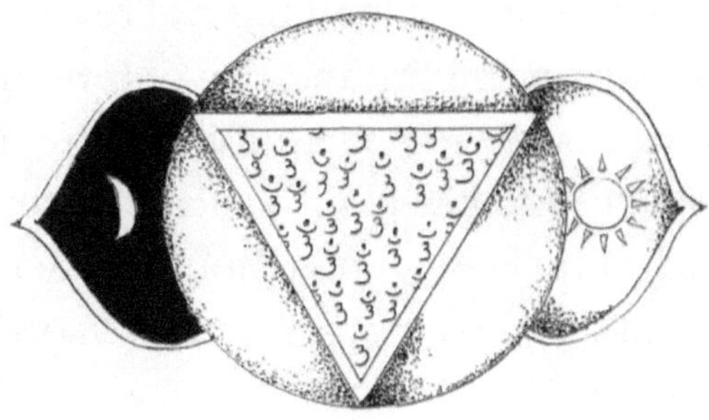

The symbol for this chakra has two lotus petals signifying the moon and the sun.

The inverted triangle in the middle is for Shakti – described as the primordial cosmic energy responsible for the dynamic nature of the universe.

Signs of imbalance in the Third Eye chakra

Physical signs

Our Western culture has been dismissive of spiritual or psychic experiences since the industrial revolution, or arguably the witch burnings and rise of formal religions where access to God is only via the church or a priest. The subsequent lack of use has led it to atrophy somewhat – in comparison to animals who. it is thought use the pineal gland to communicate so they can move as one in a shoal or flock.

The gland is subject to calcification when fluoride is consumed (added to most toothpastes and water in some countries) so a lot of people develop a hard shell around the gland which makes it harder to access its spiritual function. This can be treated by taking apple cider vinegar or iodine supplements, as well as avoiding fluoride in water or toothpaste.

Problems in the third eye chakra may also be reflected in vision challenges in our anatomical eyes, migraines and headaches, earache, blocked sinuses.

Emotional and Psychological signs

As the eye of the soul, a lack of energy or blockage around this chakra, can lead to confusion, uncertainty and pessimism. Not to mention a lack of spiritual connection.

In extreme cases this might show up as psychotic incidents and an inability to distinguish between what we refer to as reality and other perceptions.

Supporting your third eye chakra

Yoga support

(See supporting video on youtube.com/catherineshovlin)

Third Eye Awareness

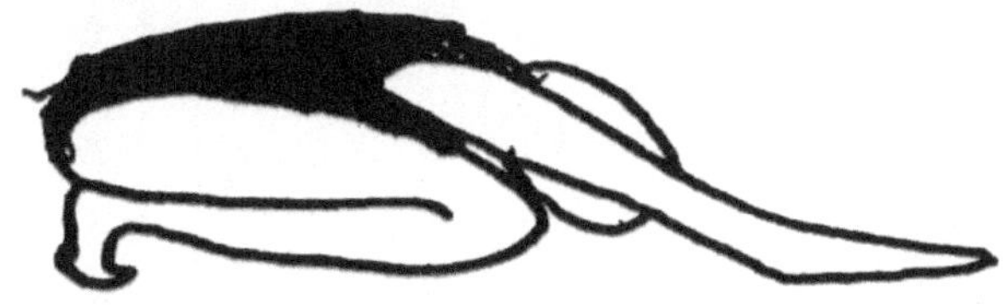

The simplest way to bring energy to this chakra is to rest in child's pose. This means kneeling on a mat, then bringing your bottom down to rest on your heels. If that isn't easy for you, then try slipping a small cushion between them. If you

How: ...Third eye chakra

suffer from pain in your knees you might also want to have some padding under them.

Then lift up as you inhale, exhaling as you fold deeply from the hips.

You may be able to rest your forehead on the ground. If not, then you can use a yoga block or your palms or fists to support it. It is important that you feel this gentle pressure on your forehead.

Now breathe slowly and deeply, noticing how the posture pushes your breath towards the back of your lungs. Close your eyes and relax. Stay here for at least a couple of minutes.

Eye Opening

In palming we cover our anatomical eyes, relaxing them and bringing attention to the third eye chakra between our eyebrows.

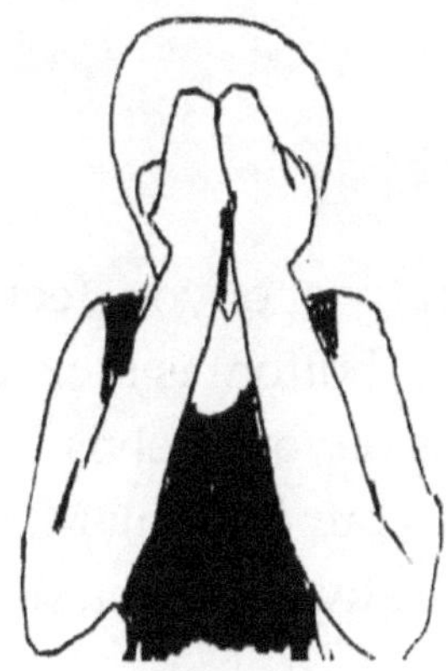

Sit comfortably and rub the palms of your hands together vigorously, to generate heat.

Then place your hands over your eyes, cupping them slightly to close out any light.

Feel the warmth of your hands soaking into your eyes, relaxing all the tiny muscles in the eye socket and the eye itself.

Feel the positive energy soaking into your eyes and the spaciousness between your eyebrows as the third eye chakra is energized by the pose.

Third Eye Reaching

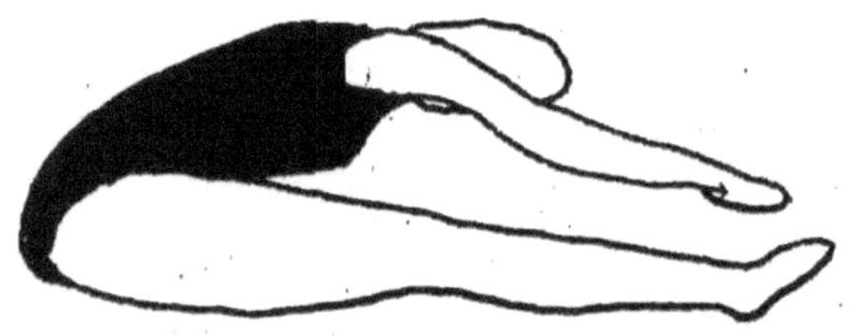

Seated on the mat, stretch your legs out in front of you, feet flexed (pointing up to the sky). Check your bottom is tucked behind you so you are sitting on the bones of your pelvis ("sit bones") and not on the fleshy part of your bottom. Most of us need to reach under and move the fleshy part back so feel free to do that.

Now inhale and reach up towards the sky with your arms, noticing how that lifts your rib cage and creates space.

As you exhale, fold forward from the hips, focusing on reaching forward rather than down. No forcing here, we want to protect our lower back.

If your forehead can rest comfortably on your legs, then sit like that. It is important to have the forehead against something as we want to work on the third eye chakra so use a cushion or a block if you need to.

Stay in the pose for 5-10 slow deep breaths then inhale as you curl back up to sitting.

Third Eye Focus

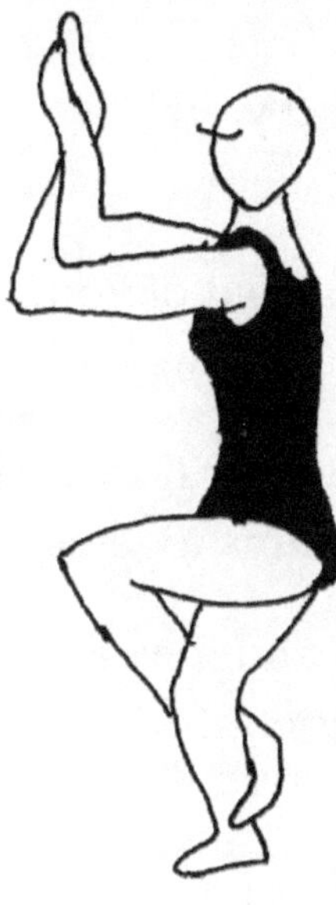

This pose can seem a bit confusing if it's your first time, though it is actually easier to do than to explain!

Stand on your mat with your feet a few centimeters apart. Find a spot on the floor, a few meters in front of you, so you can focus on it. This will help you balance.

Take your weight onto your right foot so that you can start to lift your left foot off the ground.

Raise your left knee until your thigh is parallel to the floor, letting your foot hang down.

Now tuck your left foot round the back of your right leg, as though you were crossing your knees on a bar stool.

How: …Third eye chakra

If you can, bring your left foot all the way round the back of your leg to face forwards, that's great.

Keep breathing slowly and steadily as you find your balance.

When you are ready, stretch both arms out in front of you and cross the right arm over the left above the elbow.

Bend both arms so your hands move towards your nose and cross them again at the wrists to bring your palms together.

Keep your upper arms parallel to the ground and look at your spot with all the calm focus of an eagle identifying its prey.

See if you can take 5 slow breaths in the full pose.

When you are ready, slowly unwind your arms and release them back down to your sides, then unwind your legs and return to standing.

Repeat on the other side.

Notice how this posture increases your focus and sense of clarity.

How: ...Third eye chakra

Third Eye Breath

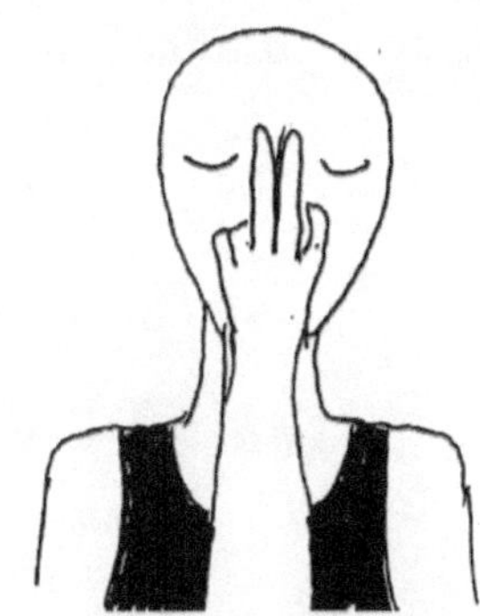

Sit in a comfortable position and hold your right hand in front of your face, with the palm facing you.

Fold down your third and fourth finger then rest your first and second finger between your eyebrows on your third eye. You should find that your thumb is resting by your right nostril and your third finger by your left.

Inhale and exhale twice through both nostrils. Start with the right nostril if you wish to energize and the left if you wish to calm yourself.

Let's say you wish to energize.

Use your third finger to close your left nostril and inhale through your right. Exhale to your right then use your thumb to close your right nostril and open the left one. Inhale and exhale through this nostril.

Continue to alternate in this manner, slowly and calmly. With your gaze centered on your third eye.

How: …Third eye chakra

If you are using this breath to calm yourself for example before going to sleep, you could do a few rounds of using only the left nostril for inhaling and exhaling as that calms the nervous system.

Supporting activities

Third Eye Journaling

As the third eye chakra connects to our intuition it is interesting to use it in this way.

Ideally do your journaling first thing in the morning, before you are completely wide awake. I keep mine by my bed and sit up to write in it. I don't put the light on.

The key to this style of journaling is that you keep writing. At first you might just write "I don't know what to write, I have nothing to say" and so on. It doesn't matter. Keep going. Repeat yourself. Spell things wrong. Talk gibberish. You might include remembered snatches of dreams. Things you woke up thinking about. How you are feeling, physically and emotionally. You might find that you have written an opinion you didn't realize you had, or a decision that you didn't even know you had made.

Let the words pour out of you. Don't stop to edit yourself. This is not for anybody but you. Let it flow. When you have finished, you might want to notice anything surprising that came up. I know this happens for me. I surprise or even shock myself sometimes. But it is nearly always my truth.

Third Eye Vision board

You may have made a vision board in the past, at a workshop maybe or as a New Year ritual. I've noticed sometimes when there are several people in a room doing that, the way they might sneak a look at each other's. Or a hand might reach out for an image and then check itself and pull back.

So, this time, do it in private and give your intuition free rein. This isn't about your strategy or manifesting or achieving goals. This is a peek into your own subconscious.

As you settle to the task, promise yourself there will be no judgment, no self-editing, no preconceptions, no shame.

Have a big enough sheet of paper – or your bedroom wall. And a pile of magazines or images from books that you don't mind tearing out. Throw in a few headlines from newspapers too so you have a word bank.

Try to think as little as possible as you let your hand pick up whatever words or pictures it is drawn to. You don't need to make sense of it at this stage. Just gather your treasure, the images that catch your eye or the words that resonate.

How: ...Third eye chakra

When you have your pile, sit with it for a moment just breathing and accepting it. Shuffle the pieces around a bit and see what emerges.

If you had to tell a short story referring to what is in front of you what might you say? You could be surprised at the insights that you come up with.

You may want to stick the pictures on the paper or your wall as a reminder. I am often amazed when I revisit a vision board like this a year later and recognized the way the images have become reality.

Sound support

You can also hum or chant to attune the third eye chakra. The Sanskrit sound for the sacral chakra is AUM (pronounced Om) and the note on the Western (diatonic) scale is A.

And as always, check out the sound tracks available online to tune into this chakra. You could play one while you are doing the vision board exercise above.

Nutritional support

Foods that support this chakra include those on the dark blue / purple spectrum like aubergine (eggplant), black grapes and purple varieties of kale, cabbage, carrots or sweet potatoes.

How: ...Third eye chakra

You might also be able to get hold of blue-green algae at your local health food store.

Foods rich in Omega 3 (good for brain) are also helpful eg salmon, avocado, flaxseed, most nuts.

And for the sweet toothed among you, a moderate amount of dark chocolate (preferably organic and fair trade) will deliver feel good hormone serotonin while nourishing your third eye chakra.

Recipe for Visionary Salad

Ingredients (per person)

- 1 handful of purple kale
- ½ eggplant (aubergine)
- 2 purple carrots
- Some purple sprouting broccoli
- Pine nuts
- 1 handful black grapes

For the dressing:

- 1 tablespoon of raisins
- 1 teaspoon honey
- 1 tablespoon of extra virgin olive oil
- ½ teaspoon sumac or some lemon zest
- 1 garlic clove, finely minced or put through a garlic press
- Juice of half a lemon

How: …Third eye chakra

- Seasoning to taste

Instructions

1. Mix all the dressing ingredients together in a small cup so the raisins have a chance to soak a little while you prepare the rest.
2. Dry fry the pine nuts for a minute or so till they are turning brown. Keep tossing them because they turn very suddenly. Set them aside to cool off.
3. Chop the carrots and eggplant (aubergine) into small cubes
4. Heat a tablespoonful of your favorite healthy oil over a medium heat in a large frying pan or wok.
5. Add the carrots and stir fry for 2-3 minutes.
6. Add the eggplant (aubergine) and continue to stir fry for a couple of minutes.
7. Turn down the heat a little and cook for 5-10 minutes more
8. Chop the broccoli into bite size florets and cut the stems into 5mm slices. Add to the frying pan or wok and keep stir frying everything until the broccoli is al dente.
9. Turn off the heat and allow to cool for a few minutes.
10. Meanwhile tear the kale into pieces the size that you like to eat and toss in a large salad bowl with half the dressing and the vegetables from the frying pan.
11. Slice the grapes in two and remove any pips.

12. Serve in bowls topped with grapes and pine nuts and with the remaining dressing in a small jug. See what visions you can conjure up while you are eating it!

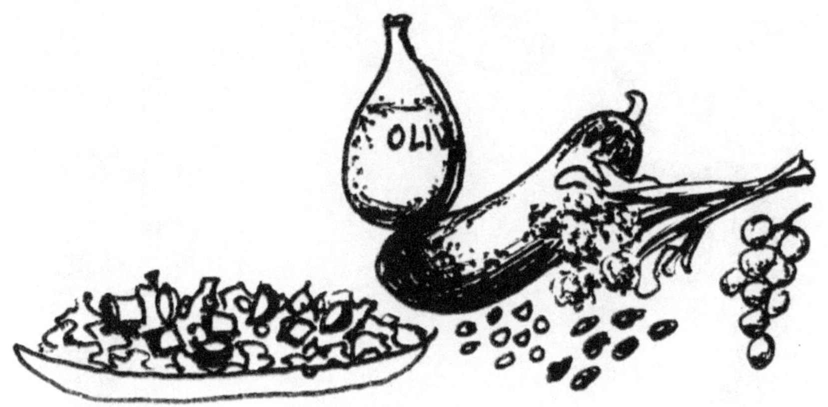

Crown chakra

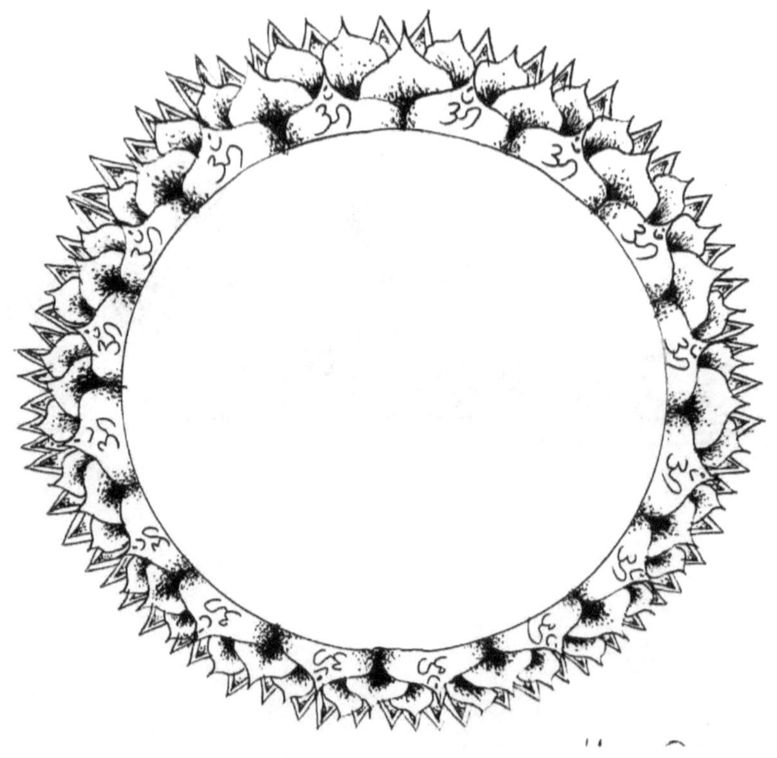

Information about the crown chakra

Introduction

This highest of the seven chakras we are exploring is actually just above the body, hovering over the crown of your head. It's no coincidence that it is in the place where a halo would be depicted in a religious painting.

It can also be considered to be at the crown of the head. If you have cared for a newborn baby, you probably know about the fontanelle. That soft spot on the skull that helps the birthing process and closes usually in the first one or two months of the baby's life. That is where the crown chakra is, and in some cultures, it is considered to be open at birth because the baby is still very connected to the wider universe, to the beyond.

The turban, or nowadays in the West, the classic yoga top knot, are thought by some to protect this chakra and to act as antenna to bring in spiritual energy.

The physical aspects related to this chakra are around the head – especially the most recently evolved part of our brain, the cerebral cortex. This covers the outside of our brain, providing connection between different aspects and giving us insights, analysis, decision making, intelligence, the ability to make conscious choices, making meaning of the information coming from our senses - what we see, hear, touch, smell and taste.

The crown chakra is related to the concept of a belief system that involves some kind of higher power – including but not limited to formal religions.

As well as religions, this chakra might be evidenced in a belief such as in the power of nature, of collective intelligence, of human spirit, of astrology, or of quantum physics. Any sense that there is something beyond the here and now, the immediately apparent. A bigger picture.

Color

The color of this chakra is violet – you can also consider it as bright white light. This is the highest vibration color that the human eye can normally see. It is the innermost color on the rainbow.

Beyond that on the electro-magnetic spectrum we have ultra-violet light – about 10% of sunlight and the part that causes us sunburn. You may also have seen ultra-violet being used to sterilize as it interacts with organic matter. It is not visible to most humans, but it can be seen by insects, birds and some mammals. The beneficial effect for us of UVB rays in sunlight is the formation of Vitamin D in our bodies – essential for life and a trigger for the production of feel-good hormone serotonin in our bodies.

Expand your senses with high vibration violet or pure white light. Feel your spirit lift to it and float away in the ether.

Element

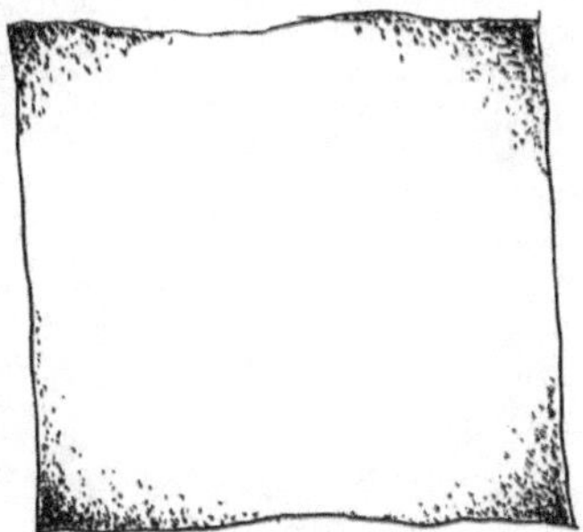

As with the throat and third eye chakras, the element for the crown chakra is ether. Maybe more than any other chakra it gives us a wide connection with the universe, all the people, beings, planets, stars, trees, mountains... and all the space in between. The cosmic energy that powers our universe.

When you consider the 7 chakras in a column from your tailbone to the crown of your head, you might also envision the energy from the crown chakra fanning out in all directions like an exceptionally bright candle.

Name and Symbol

The Sanskrit name for the crown chakra – *Sahasrara* – represents the connection point between heaven and earth. Between the feminine, *Shakti* energy rising through us from the earth and the masculine *Shiva* energy coming down from the sky. The connection between us as individuals and us as unity.

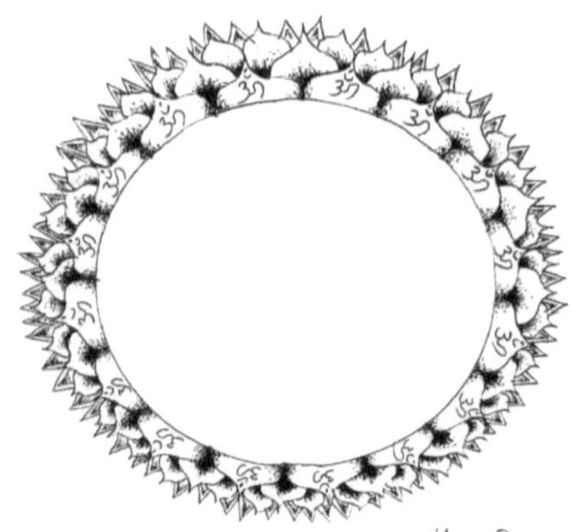

The crown chakra is symbolized by the 1000 petalled lotus. At its center is a simple circle – the void, the ether – and around it a multitude of petals to represent the 1000 that would take a long time to draw.

The essence of this chakra is the spaciousness and expansion of the universe – and therefore our own being. Imagine a flower over the crown of your head opening and opening and opening, more and more petals curling open and shining their bright white light over you.

Signs of imbalance in the crown chakra

Physical signs

Because the crown chakra is related to the brain, it is connected to chronic brain related issues such as frequent incapacitating headaches and ongoing degenerative conditions like Parkinson's or Alzheimer's.

More acutely, accidents or illnesses causing brain damage often affect our personality and moods and can cause depression, physical limitations and ultimately death.

On a more day to day level, headaches and insomnia may result from a disturbed energy field around this chakra.

Remembering that the crown chakra is connected to our interpretation of sensory information, a sign of imbalance can also be if we lose sensitivity – responsiveness to our senses.

We may find ourselves no longer enjoying our food, or not seeing the beauty of the world around us – either physically or metaphorically. Becoming numb or desensitized in any way.

Emotional and Psychological signs

Low energy in the crown chakra can be associated with a loss of faith – this may be in human nature, in yourself or the people around you as well as losing faith in your religion.

How: …Crown chakra

You may also find yourself struggling to see the bigger picture or failing to find your place in society.

Becoming overly focused on the needs of the ego or the small-self indicate you may have issues around crown chakra energy, as do frequently experiencing boredom and seeking stimulus all the time. This tendency can also manifest as greediness, grasping for everything in the hope to fill the void inside.

A tendency to extreme or addictive actions can be observed - even around 'good' things like exercise, fasting or meditating. Others can become addicted to specific gurus or teachers, losing their ability for discernment or judgment, and accepting everything the guru or teacher says as absolute fact. This could be dangerous in a cult type situation.

We all need to find ways to hold on to our sense of self and the world.

So, be aware of imbalances in this area and take steps to make the necessary adjustments. Be in your own power – not the way outside forces think you should be, not a poor copy of someone else's power- but your very own unique set of experiences, skills and characteristics.

Supporting your crown chakra

Yoga support

(See supporting video on youtube.com/catherineshovlin)

Meditation

The best kind of yoga for the crown chakra is meditation. If you already have a practice, then you might give it a crown chakra focus for a few days and see what changes you notice.

If you have never meditated, it may be one of those things you feel you "can't do" or maybe can't be bothered with. I hear people explain to me that their mind is too busy, and they can't turn it off.

I invite you to let go of these limiting beliefs about meditation and yourself.

Often the *intention* of emptying your mind, which is indeed part of meditation, is seen as the goal. The target. So, we try to do that and of course fail, because our human mind is a hotbed of thoughts, memories, ideas, responses. That leads to a sense of failure or getting disheartened.

Our waking mind needs to be alert and responsive; it is just doing its job of keeping us alive. Think of the aim rather as smoothing out what is going on in your mind. Shifting to a different frequency. Retuning the radio.

Everybody has meditated, even if they haven't labelled it as such. Maybe when being 'in the flow' during a sporting activity, or totally absorbed and present in the moment. It is a state of brainwave activity. Our brainwaves operate at 4 different ranges. Although all 4 can be present at the same time, we tend to classify our state by the dominant brainwave patterns.

- **Beta** (15-40 cycles per second): This is our regular workaday state when we are awake. Lots going on. Maybe multitasking. Doing one thing while worrying about another. Alert, responsive, reactive. It can also be a state of anxiety or depression, especially if we don't give ourselves a break from it. When we are dreaming or in the REM sleeping stage, we can also be in this state if the dreams put us into an active mode.
- **Alpha** (9-14 cycles per second): A brain at rest. A more spacious brain state, good for creativity, ideas, learning. Relieves depression. As we start to meditate or fall asleep, we also go into this state. We may experience vivid imagery and feel very open to what might be possible.
- **Theta:** (5-8 cycles per second): Associated with daydreaming, hypnosis or that state where you realise you just arrived somewhere without remembering the drive there. Running in nature or taking a shower might get you there. Being in this state improves our chemistry by reducing cortisol and increasing feel good chemicals like serotonin.

How: …Crown chakra

> Meditating can also bring us to this state. If you are asleep in this state you are usually dreaming, even if you don't remember it.
>
> - **Delta:** (1-5-4 cycles per second). Extremely deep meditation or dreamless sleep. Also experienced in Stage 1 sleep. A state where our immune system is strengthened, and healing takes place.

So, by meditating we mean our brain is awake yet relaxed. We are not fretting, analyzing, overthinking, concentrating, learning or trying to work anything out.

For many people it can help to get into this state if they focus on one thing rather than trying to think of nothing. Focusing on your breathing is a great tool for meditation since it is so readily accessible.

Become aware of your breathing without interfering with it. Let it carry on naturally, though breathe through your nose if you can as that calms the nervous system. Feel the slight rush of cool air as it enters your nostrils, and the softer ebb of warmer air as you exhale.

Just sit still and do this for a minute or two. The more you can keep your body still, the easier it will be for your mind to still.

Notice how you feel different. Calmer maybe. More focused and alert? Less stressed or overwhelmed?

That was you meditating.

How: ...Crown chakra

If you like the feeling and want to do more of it, then you may find it useful to follow one of the many apps and online programs now available. Try a few different teaching methods and go with the one that feels most aligned to you and your brain characteristics. See if you can stick to it for a week.

If that goes ok, then try another week.

The aim is not to DO meditation like doing the laundry or playing a soccer match. It's more like ALLOWING it to happen. You don't need to admonish yourself for not meditating "properly". Just observe what happens, with compassion. It is one meditation in a sea of meditations. The next one will be different. Every one that you do will be different.

One of the great things I find is that if I meditate regularly (this regularity seems to make more difference than the amount of time I do it for), and especially if I sit in the same place, ideally at the same time of day to do it, then my physical body starts to recognize the cues and it becomes easier to get into a meditative state.

Accept the ups and downs of meditation. It's not like doing press ups where you will automatically get better and better. Stick at it and I hope that, like me, you will find it gives you more equanimity with life's ups and downs, less susceptibility to mood swings and even moments of pure joy.

How: …Crown chakra

For those used to longer meditations, look online for a recording of the Melting Ointment or Melting Butter meditation. This is particularly powerful for the crown chakra.

Crown Chakra Awareness

If you can manage it, a headstand is a wonderful stimulus for the crown chakra. Please make sure you are safe and sufficiently experienced to do that posture and only go as far as you feel strong and stable.

If you don't feel that is for you – and I for one do not! - then try this modified version. You will get a lot of the same benefits… and maybe one day you'll find your legs just float up to the sky!

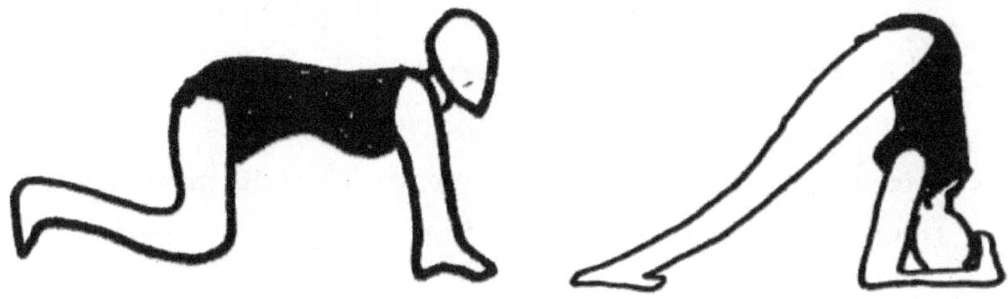

Start on all fours, hands under your shoulders, knees under your hips.

Take a few breaths and calmly state your intention to bring awareness to your crown chakra for greater connection to the universe. You might want to offer up the practice to a person or a situation that is troubled.

How: …Crown chakra

Go down onto your elbows and hold opposite elbows with your hands. This will make sure your arms are correctly spaced.

Without moving your elbows, move your forearms forward so you can clasp your hands. You are making a triangular base for your posture. To make sure the sides of both hands are securely grounded, curl in the lowest finger. Raise your thumbs towards the sky.

Now lower your head so that the top of your head is on the floor and the back of your head is snugly against the support of your hands. This might be enough for you. Stay here for 5-10 slow deep breaths, bringing your energy to your crown chakra and your connection to the earth and all that live on it.

If you want to go a bit further, curl your toes under, start to straighten your legs and lift up your tailbone like you would in downward dog. Check your alignment. You want your neck to feel comfortable and your shoulders to be pulling away from your head not scrunched towards your ears.

You can start to walk your feet towards your head. If you spend a minute or two on this each day, you will find that you become more comfortable with the posture and can go a little further or stay a little longer each time.

When you feel you have completed, slowly lower your knees back down to the mat, release your head, release your arms and sit back on your heels for a few breaths to settle.

Wake Up your Crown Chakra

This posture feels good at the end of your yoga practice, or on its own when you've been having a demanding day and feel like your head is buzzing with too many thoughts.

Sit comfortably and make loose fists with your hands. Shake your arms a bit to loosen your shoulders, elbows and wrists.

Inhale as you raise your arms above your head then exhale as you lower them to your skull and start to very gently pound your head with your knuckles. Use your intuition to guide you as to the right amount of pressure… it certainly shouldn't give you any discomfort.

Keep your shoulders and jaw relaxed and breathe calmly and steadily.

Keep gently rapping your skull for a few minutes.

You can explore how it feels different on the top or sides of your head. Take good care of yourself. The aim is to stimulate blood flow to the scalp (good for hair growth too!) and release some of the trapped energy from our Western tendency to get "stuck in our head" all the time.

Finish by reaching up into the sky and using your fingertips to pour gentle "rain" from the crown of your head all the way down your body.

How: …Crown chakra

Deep relaxation

This may not seem like a posture at all, but in fact it is one of the most important in your yoga practice.

Lie on your back on the mat.

Take a couple of deep slow breaths into your belly. Continue to breathe in and out through your nose if you can, your mouth if you need to.

Pull your knees towards your chest to release your lower back and then lower your legs one at a time to the mat, feet hip distance apart and falling slightly outwards in a relaxed way.

Have your arms by your sides, palms facing upwards, slightly away from your body so they are not touching your torso.

Check that the back of your neck is long, chin slightly tucked.

Take a couple of deeper breaths, exhaling through your mouth with a sigh.

Now scan your body, starting at the right foot. Let's focus on our connections – the joints in our body.

Relax all the small joints in the toes of your right foot, and your ankle. Relax your right knee and then your hip.

Relax all the small joints in the toes of your left foot, and your left ankle. Relax your left knee and then your hip.

How: …Crown chakra

Relax your tailbone where it joins your sacrum, and all the vertebrae up your spine. Run your attention up your spine from bottom to top, feeling each vertebra settle into the mat.

Relax all the small joints in the fingers of your right hand, and your wrist. Relax your right elbow and then your shoulder.

Relax all the small joints in the fingers of your left hand, and your left wrist. Relax your left elbow and then your shoulder.

Relax the connections between your shoulders and your collar bones and shoulder blades.

Relax the back of your neck where it joins your skull.

Relax your jaw where it connects to your skull.

And relax your face muscles too.

Smooth your forehead.

Relax your cheeks. Relax all the tiny muscles around your eyes and your eyebrows.

Imagine you are relaxing the tiny muscle of each eyelash.

Relax your teeth and your tongue. Let the tip of your tongue rest against the ridge just behind your top teeth.

Relax your abdomen and all of your organs. Let them settle into the ground and breathe peacefully.

How: …Crown chakra

Know that the more you relax, the more you can get the benefit from the yoga you have just done. Allowing your body to integrate all the stretching and strengthening.

Know that the more you relax, the more you can nourish your sense of well-being.

When you feel you have completed your relaxation, start to breathe a little more deeply.

Bring your awareness to your fingers and toes and wriggle them.

Circle your wrists and ankles.

When you are ready, roll over onto your right side. Take a couple of deep breaths here and then bring yourself back to a seated position. Your practice is complete.

How: …Crown chakra

Supporting activities

Being

The best way to support this chakra is not by DOING anything but rather by practicing BEING.

Mindfulness, meditation and simple activities like walking, coloring in and knitting all soothe your brainwaves and are a good tonic for this chakra.

For the last couple of years, I have been in Bali for NYEPI – their new year festival, usually sometime in late March. For an entire day the island is dark. No internet, no telephone or TV. No vehicles on the roads or planes in the sky. Factories and offices are closed. Everybody stays home to contemplate.

In 2019 this seemed like an exceptional state of affairs. However, in 2020 with the COVID-19 experience, it is much more familiar to us.

The next day I felt cleansed. Like a reset. I also made more conscious choices after that about how I did want to engage with the activities that usually feel almost essential. But of course are not, they are mostly just habits.

The idea of a whole day DOING nothing might be alarming. It helps a lot that during NYEPI everyone around is in the same situation, but the experience is something you could recreate for yourself.

Imagine a whole day of no social media, no internet browsing, no checking your phone, no Netflix, no work, no busyness. I found that I might spend an entire hour watching raindrops dripping from a leaf, or ants going about their work.

Drumming

Activities that stop the chatter in our minds are supportive for the crown chakra.

Try something a bit new to you like drumming or working with gongs.

Let yourself be absorbed into the activity, coming at it from your body and intuition rather than your brain. This is not a performance and your technical capacity to drum is of no consequence. Let yourself go into the activity and drop any attachment to a good musical outcome.

You may feel yourself switch so that it seems the drum is playing you rather than the other way around.

Afterwards you may feel delightfully fatigued, or totally refreshed. Like the garden after a rainstorm.

Aromatherapy

Frankincense is a good oil for the crown chakra. Try some in an essential oil vaporizer while you meditate. Or add it to oil and rub it on your aptly named temples.

How: ...Crown chakra

Breathe in slowly and deeply, imagining that the frankincense is cleansing your brain of unwanted thoughts.

Sound support

You can also hum or chant to attune the crown chakra. The Sanskrit sound for the crown chakra is OM and the note on the Western scale is B.

Humming can be particularly powerful for the crown chakra. You do not need to hum any particular tune or note, just let each exhalation be a hum. This is sometimes referred to as Bee Breath. Maybe it should be called Be Breath!

You may be able to feel the vibration tuning up your receptivity to higher energies.

Nutritional support

If you are working deeply with the crown chakra, you may feel that food is a distraction and fasting is more appropriate. Listen to your body and do what feels right. For the last few months I have been doing gentle intermittent fasting – 14 hours of not eating and a 10-hour period when I can eat. As well as noticing a significant decrease in my urge to snack, and a good improvement in my body's management of blood sugar levels, I also feel I am more able to focus and think clearly. You might want to give it a try!

If on the other hand you feel you need to tempt yourself a little to eat, then try liquid foods and light meals.

Recipe for easy chia dessert

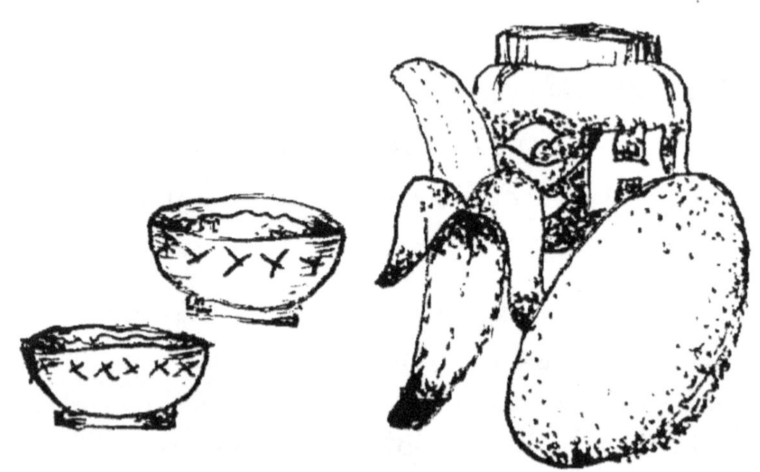

I like to have a couple of these in the fridge for moments when I fancy something to eat but don't feel like a proper meal. It's cool and refreshing and slips down easily – as well as being nourishing of course. It takes minutes to make and can last up to a week in the fridge.

Chia seeds are a gluten-free superfood prized by the Mayans and so highly thought of that they were offered to the gods by the Aztecs thousands of years ago.

They are rich in antioxidants and also offer you fiber, iron, manganese, magnesium and calcium. They are a good source of protein, containing all nine essential amino acids that cannot be made by our own bodies - especially valuable for those following a plant-based diet.

Crown chakra

Depending on the fruit you use you will get the benefits from that too. Soaking the seeds in this way makes them easier to digest and easier for the body to extract nutrition.

This simple technique also creates an interesting texture as the seeds absorb ten times their own volume in liquid.

Ingredients (per portion)

- A teaspoonful of chia seeds
- Half a cup of fruit juice. I like mango but feel free to experiment. Because this is crown chakra you might want to use the juice of a white fruit like apple, pear or guava.
- Toppings (optional) eg thinly sliced banana, cacao nibs, pomegranate seeds, granola

Instructions

1. Couldn't be easier! Stir the seeds into the juice and leave in the fridge for a few hours or overnight.
2. Add any toppings that feel right in the moment, grab a spoon and tuck in.
3. As well as being great to eat on its own, you can use this as a topping on ice cream or other desserts crying out for some of its juicy fruitiness.

Crown chakra

Choose the chakra you want to focus on for the day and slip the appropriately colored stone into your pocket. At various points in the day you might come across it and, prompted by the color, breathe into that chakra a few times. Even when you don't do that, know that the stone is there in your pocket, working for you and with you.

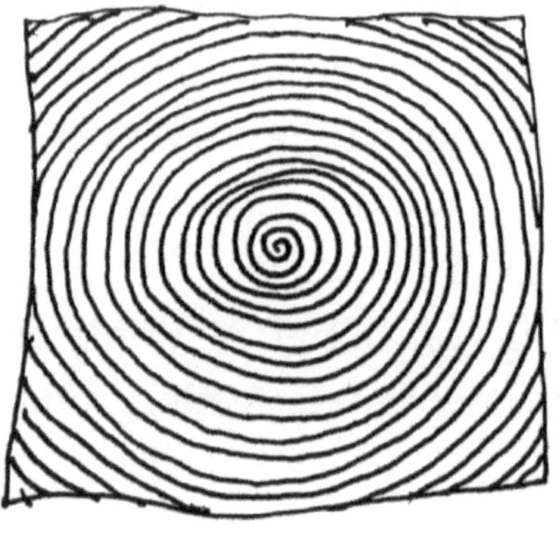

Integration

Part 3: integrating chakras to live life in full color

Your chakra journey

Knowing about chakras is just the beginning of your lifelong journey with these powerful energy centers. I hope that what I have shared with you has piqued your interest in understanding and working with your chakras so you can live in full color.

There is an abundance of more detailed information on meditations, music, yoga, foods and so on available online or in your bookstore. Or you might prefer a more internal journey, working with what you have learnt here and your own intuition or access to collective wisdom.

Remember that at some level you already know everything you need to know. For example, you might be feeling more tired than usual. Unconsciously your hand moves to your throat and gently massages your throat chakra, stimulating your thyroid and metabolic function. You don't need to know what happened, you just have to notice what your body is calling for and follow the instinct. That is enough for some people.

Others prefer to have a more detailed understanding of what is happening and why. Luckily both routes – and many other variations – are available to you.

My hope with this information is that it gives you opportunities to feel more alive – as it has for me. To step up from a black and white existence into living in full color.

And to know how to finetune the balance so you feel at ease and ready for life.

Chakra Integration

I encourage you to consider all of the chakras as aspects of one system. You would expect to see all the colors in a rainbow, not have some missing. By working with your chakras as a whole system, or whole spectrum of possibilities, you will be able to balance your energies and address any blockages.

A common pitfall is to have a sense that higher chakras are more worthy or important than lower chakras. In fact, if we are too much in the higher chakras at the expense of our root, sacral and solar plexus chakras, we might become heady, ungrounded, a little unstable.

The best situation is a harmonious full range. A complete rainbow. That gives us the basis we need for a fulfilling life. A life in full color

The following suggestions can be a good starting practice to develop this.

Chakra scan

Sit comfortably with your spine straight and your feet firmly on the floor (or cross legged on a mat if you prefer). Inhale and exhale slowly and gently three times to be sure you are fully present.

(See supporting video on youtube.com/catherineshovlin)

Integration…Your chakra journey

Round 1 - location

As you do this round, notice which chakras feel "easy" and which are more elusive. No judgement or correction is required, just notice.

On the next inhale, imagine you are inhaling through your root chakra, at the base of your spine, bringing energy to it. Exhale through your root chakra.

Then inhale and exhale through your sacral chakra.

Do this with each chakra in turn (solar plexus, heart, throat, third eye, crown) imagining each time that the breath is coming into and going out of your body through that chakra.

Round 2 - color

Go through the breathing cycle of round 1 again, this time adding in the color for each chakra.

Inhale through your root chakra and imagine the color red emanating from that point, blooming softly into the surrounding area like a drop of ink in water.

Do the same for the sacral chakra with the color orange. And then each in turn:

- Solar plexus – yellow

- Heart – green

- Throat – aqua

- Third eye – indigo

- Crown – violet

By now you may be starting to feel the buzz of the breath and the chakras as they activate

Round 3 - sound

For the last round let's add sound.

So still considering the location and the color of each chakra, now include the sound. Don't worry if you don't know exactly what a note sounds like. Just follow your instincts and the general principle of going up a notch with each successive chakra.

As a reminder, the notes and sounds are listed in the table below. You can either just sing or hum the note or use the sounds as well.

Chakra	Color	Note	Sound
Root	Red	C	LAM (pronounced lomm)
Sacral	Orange	D	VAM (pronounced vomm)
Solar plexus	Yellow	E	RAM (pronounced romm)

Integration…Your chakra journey

Heart	Green	F	YAM (pronounced yomm)
Throat	Aqua	G	HAM (pronounced homm)
Third eye	Indigo	A	OM
Crown	Violet	B	OM

Once you are familiar with this sequence, the whole thing will take 2-3 minutes to complete. And it will get easier to hold the different aspects in mind at the same time.

Each time you repeat these three rounds, you are helping your body remember these energy centers and giving therapeutic attention to each one of them.

Maybe one day you observe in Round 1 that your throat chakra is tight. Is there something you haven't been saying? Are you being true to yourself? By the end of the exercise, it may well have cleared, so you can now feel the energy flowing freely up and down your body.

Another day it may be your heart chakra that's in a tangle, or your third eye chakra that's totally overstimulated.

Remember not to judge any of these things. Observe them. Accept them. Love them if you can. You will often find they have shifted – maybe dissolved or feel more balanced by the end of the 3 rounds.

Flip it!

The previous exercise is designed to tune up the chakras. It will energize you and can give you a feeling of clarity and even ecstasy.

At other times you may want to calm and ground yourself for instance before sleeping or after an emotional upset. In this case follow the same process but for each round start at the crown chakra and work your way down to the root chakra.

Using chakras diagnostically

Because different organs and areas of the body relate to different chakras, you might know that one area is more frequently challenged for you either physically or emotionally. That could be blocked, or under-powered or over-stimulated.

Having identified a specific chakra that you wish to work on and give more love and support to, look through the activities suggested in that chapter and select something that appeals to you. Or find music online designed to heal that chakra and listen to it while you meditate or relax.

You can use the colors too of course. Try wearing the color of the chakra you want to stimulate, or the opposite to the color that is overstimulated (red is the opposite to green, blue is the opposite to orange, yellow is the opposite to violet). Or surround yourself with that color.

Next time you change your duvet cover or select a new notebook in the stationery shop, pause for a second to think what color you need more of in your life. Which chakra needs a bit more support right now? Or which one will help you most in that activity?

Stand up for chakras!

Imagine that each of your chakras is a spinning sphere. When you sit or stand with a straight spine, they can balance more easily one on top of the other.

On the other hand, if for instance we tend to curl over our tummy because we feel embarrassed about it, or hunch over our heart to protect it, the spheres are no longer balanced.

Try imagining this stack of spheres from your tailbone to the crown of your head and adjust your posture so you feel that they are well aligned. That means it will take less effort to keep them balanced, and the energy can flow more freely between them.

It can help to imagine you have a thread running from your tailbone up through each chakra (like beads on a string) and out of the top of your head. Feel as though you are being lifted by this string so that your upper body is almost floating over your hips.

Good posture is a habit (as is bad!). When you first increase your posture awareness it can be disheartening that you find you need to correct yourself so often. But don't worry, this is just part of the change process. The more often you notice that you have hunched over or slouched and then choose to raise yourself up, the more you are training your body in new habits.

Think of the central column of energy – the *sushumna* – as a crystal tube on which the chakra 'beads' are threaded. Keeping the tube as clean and clear as possible will help you feel stronger, more clearheaded and more energized.

Walking chakra exercise

Walking is always good for balancing our energies. It's one of my first choices when I have had an emotional upset or am feeling emotionally or creatively stuck.

As well as physical benefits, walking is also said to support the immune system, reduce stress and help with insomnia.

Because of the way female hormones work, intense physical activity can add stress chemicals to your mix, whereas gentle to moderate walking gives you exercise without increasing your stress load. This is even more true if you can walk in nature and somewhere like a beach or meadow where you don't have to think about traffic or other people and can drift into your own world.

Walking like this can be particularly helpful during hormonal turbulence around puberty, menstruation, post-partum or menopause.

Power up your walking with this chakra process.

Integration…Your chakra journey

Get into your natural relaxed rhythm - this is not a power walking moment! Notice the gentle back and forth as you put one foot in front of the other in front of the other in front of the other.

Now focus on your root chakra as you inhale for about four steps - it depends on your own natural rhythm what works best for you. Then exhale for the next four steps.

Do the same for each of the chakras in turn (sacral, solar plexus, heart, throat, third eye, crown). Finish with 4 step inhale and 4 step exhale for your whole chakra system.

When you are done, pause and notice if you feel any different. Is your walking less effort? Do you feel lighter? Or maybe your mood has changed a little?

Continue walking normally for a couple of minutes, allowing your body to integrate the balancing and clearing work you have just done. You can repeat this exercise as often as you wish.

Put your chakra in your pocket

It is a rewarding exercise to make a collection of colored chakra stones or tokens. Choose small ones that you can slip into your pocket or purse.

You might prefer the brighter colors of semi-precious stones, or the more subtle tones of pebbles you picked up on a beach. You could also use glass beads or other manufactured items, though I feel that natural objects have more power.

Integration…Your chakra journey

Each morning you can breathe through your chakras one by one, holding each stone in turn to go with the color of that chakra. (Root – red, sacral – orange, solar plexus – yellow, heart – green, throat – aqua, third eye – indigo, crown – violet). Use this exercise see which chakra feels the least comfortable, the least free. Maybe it is blocked, or underpowered or overstimulated.

Alternatively lie on your back and place the stones on each chakra. I find this a very powerful exercise for clearing blockages and increasing my energy and sense of well-being. Just lie still for five minutes like this or use one of the chakra breathing techniques described elsewhere in this book.

The 5 Tibetan Rites

(See supporting video on youtube.com/catherineshovlin)

This yoga sequence is thought to be 2,500 years old, originating in Tibet and connected to Indian yoga. It is said that they are the secret to eternal youth. To tapping into a well-spring of energy.

From our point of view, their relevance is also that they work with all 7 of the chakras, making them a nice integration sequence for our final chapter.

The final aim is to do 21 repetitions of each exercise and to do the full sequence at least once a day. I started, and I suggest you start, by doing 3 repetitions of each and then gradually build up.

Integration…Your chakra journey

Of course, you will find some moves easier than others. That is normal. Go at your own pace, move slowly and with precision. Maybe when you get to 21 repetitions a day you will try doing 3 of each and be amazed that you ever found that a challenge!

Work with your breath, stay in flow. This is not like circuit training where you are pushing out your ten sit ups as fast as possible before dashing to the next station. This is a more considered set of movements.

 As with all the yoga and meditations in this book I am putting a video on my website windsofdiscovery.com/chakras or see my channel on youtube

Rite 1: Release control

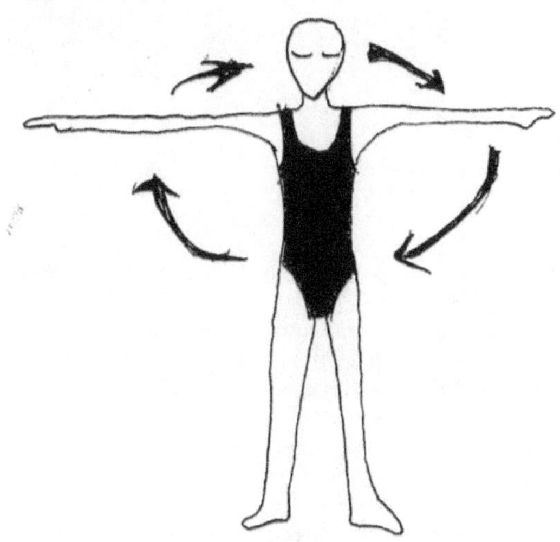

Stand with feet hip distance apart and take a breath to find your place on the earth

Exhale then as you inhale start to slowly rotate in a clockwise direction (right shoulder back, left shoulder forward), exhale as you come all the way round to face forwards again.

Do 3 repetitions.

If you suffer from severe dizziness, then slow it down. You should gradually increase your tolerance for this as you progressively increase the number of repetitions.

Accept the dizziness as part of the process. We can live with some loss of control. We can maintain our balance even when it is more difficult. We are grounded on the earth.

Rite 2: The world is your mirror

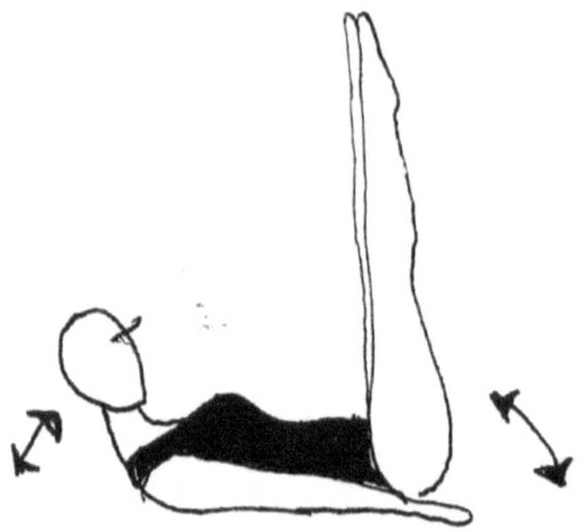

For the second move lie on your back, hands by your sides, palms down. Engage your core muscles, pulling your navel towards your spine to protect your lower back.

As you inhale raise your legs to vertical and lift your shoulders off the floor, tucking in your chin to curl your head off the floor.

As you exhale, lower your head, shoulders and legs back down to the ground.

Ideally keep your legs straight throughout. However, if you need to bend your knees while you are still working on strengthening your lower back then do so.

As you repeat this move 3 to 21 times, according to your level of progression consider that when you see the world

Integration…Your chakra journey

you see yourself. And when you see yourself you see the world.

Some days the world is a difficult place, and nothing goes our way. What is it mirroring back to us? How can we change ourselves, so we change our experience of the world?

Rite 3: As above, so below

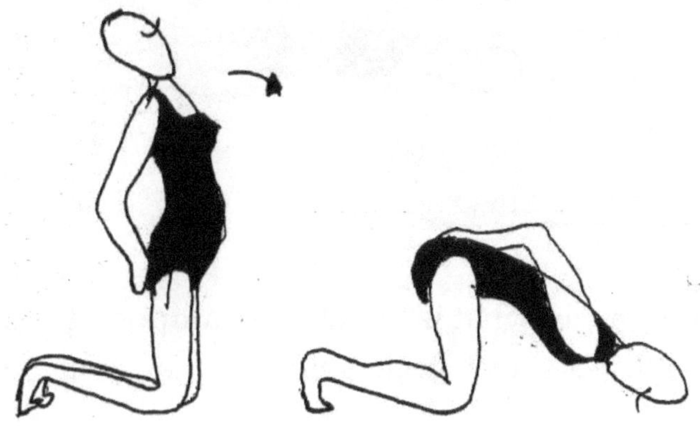

Next come on to your knees, toes tucked under, back straight, chin slightly tucked.

Place your hands firmly on the top slope of our buttocks. Keep them there throughout.

As you inhale, arch your back, look up towards the sky, head back if that is comfortable for you and your neck.

As you exhale, bow down so that your forehead touches the earth.

Inhale back up and start the next repetition.

Whatever is happening in the universe is also happening here on earth. The microcosm reflects the macrocosm. We are each part of the story and we are all connected in our intention to create heaven on earth.

Rite 4: Humility is greatness

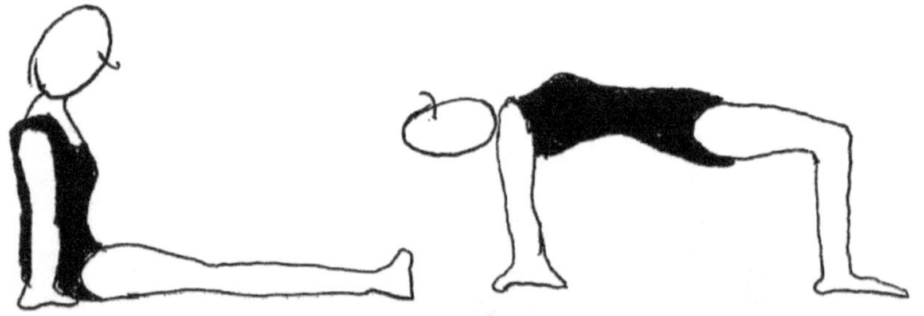

For the fourth rite start in what is known as Staff pose. Legs straight in front. Buttocks flesh back, spine straight, chin slightly tucked.

As you inhale, move your feet to be flat on the floor, raising your hips at the same time to tabletop pose. Aim for a flat alignment from your knees to the crown of your head. Clench your buttocks to support your lower back.

As you exhale, come back to the starting position.

Repeat 3 times at first, building up to 21.

Greatness is not being the most flashy or loud or self-aggrandizing. There is greatness in humility too. In putting ourselves in a position of service where we can. Offering our

Integration…Your chakra journey

gifts for the world rather than rejoicing in them to satisfy our ego.

Know your strengths so you can use them to good effect. Humility is not self-deprecation either. It is acceptance.

Rite 5: Unity

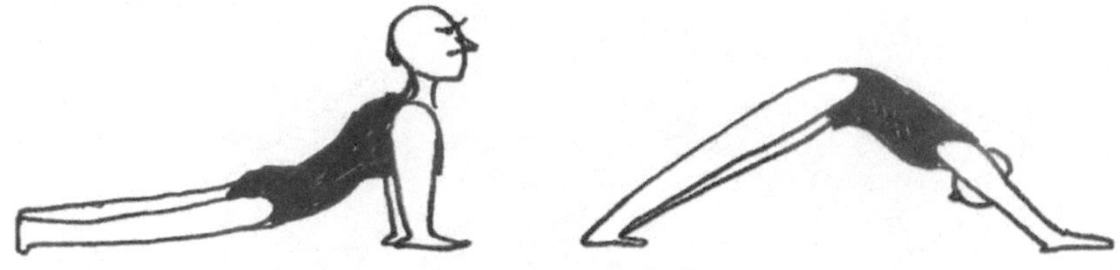

For the final move, lie on your front, hands level with your shoulders.

As you inhale, push up to straighten your arms and raise your body off the ground. Only your toes and hands are in contact with the floor. The rest of your body is suspended between your shoulders and your heels.

Check your shoulders are away from your ears and your head is raised up so you don't compress the vertebrae in the back of your neck.

As you exhale, raise your hips to create an inverted V. The pose known as downward dog.

As you go through your repetitions, notice how the body feels like it is rotating around a single point. We have unity within our body – the left side is working as hard as the right, the muscles on the back of the body are working as hard as those on the front. We have unity in our being – our mind and body are breath are working together to make this a smooth flowing movement. And maybe you can feel unity with the whole system. Our planet, our solar system, our galaxy. Unity with nature, with the sky, with the weather, with the stars. Unity with our neighbor and with someone on the other side of the world.

Closing words…

Your journey from here

Thank you for taking the time to travel with me on this journey towards living life in full color. I hope you have enjoyed the discoveries along the way. Maybe you have picked up some new habits that you might continue to use. Or some ideas for further learning and growth.

As a last little drop of information, people sometimes ask me about which aromatherapy oils work for which chakra. This is a lovely way to tune in to the one you want to work with – try a few drops in a bath, or an oil vaporizer, or mixed with a base oil to rub into your skin.

So, starting from the base, here are three suggestions for each of the chakras. You will notice that some resonate with more than one chakra – two for the price of one! It may well be that this is the perfect combination for you in a given moment. Enjoy!

- Root chakra: rich, earthy scents such as patchouli, frankincense, sandalwood
- Sacral chakra: sensual oils like ylang-ylang, jasmine, rose and neroli

- Solar plexus chakra: fresh oils including lemon, juniper and rosemary
- Heart chakra: sweet loving oils – rose, bergamot and rosewood
- Throat chakra: healing herby oils like sage, lemongrass and chamomile
- Third eye chakra: mind clearing oils including lavender, peppermint and frankincense
- Crown chakra: oils to combat disassociation and open your mind such as sandalwood, myrrh or neroli

Remember that you are all of your chakras and they are all you. It is an integrated system. From time to time you may need to put some extra focus on a particular chakra which is displaying the most signs of imbalance or which you know will have been challenged by events in your life. And we all have our tendencies to be stronger in some areas than others. Bear in mind that a chain is as strong as its weakest link so give extra support where it is needed – and consider all 7 of your chakras as an integrated system ready and willing to support you in your quest to be the best and most fulfilled version of yourself. The more you are, the more you can contribute to the world.

I know that for me, I continue to deepen my understanding of chakras and how they can help me. Each new yoga exercise that I discover, or piece of information I wasn't previously aware of enriches my understanding and my fascination with these power centers in each and every one of us. What a magnificent source of renewal and well-being.

Gratitudes

On my way to writing this book I have met many wise and wonderful teachers. Some in books and some in real life. Here are just a few of them that I would like to acknowledge and thank specifically for their contribution to my journey. They are in alphabetical order because I could not possibly rank them.

- Angela Wright who introduced me to the extraordinary power of color.
- Beth Follini who helped me realize the power of embodiment
- Cat Wheeler who guided me towards the universal wisdom we can all access
- Chiara Ramella and all the yoga teachers who showed me how to use my body to trust my instincts
- Chloe Goodchild who showed me "my wild voice sings to my power"
- Claire Zammitt who showed me how to be my true self
- Daizan Skinner Roshi who opened my eyes to the teacher within
- Fr Pat Bennett who encouraged me to do the right thing over the popular one
- Johnny Summers whose unfaltering belief in me helped me through my doubts and fears to the joy beyond

Closing words…Gratitudes

- My three extraordinary children who taught me almost all I know
- Rhiannon Augenthaler and Simon Buxton who introduced me to my guides - who were there all along waiting for me to notice them!
- The island of Bali that held me in her gentle beauty and universal connection while I wrote this book. And all of the gracious, charming, wonderful staff at Warung Lala & Lili in Ubud, Bali who kept me safe, fed, housed and inspired while I wrote.

And not forgetting all of the challenging people, the worthy opponents, that I met and have yet to meet along my journey – I won't name you here, you know who you are! – who have helped me find my strength and led me to a better understanding of my true nature.

Index :

Quickly find a specific term in the text

5 Tibetan Rites, 161
abdominal brain, 61
Acupuncture, 18
addictions, 64, 137
adult self, 91
Alpha brainwaves, 139
Anahata, 79
anger, 48
anxiety, 90
aromatherapy, 167
arrhythmia, 81
arthritis, 64
As above, so below, 164
auras, 117
ayahuasca, 115
Ayurvedic, 18
baby, 90
back problems, 33
bath, 54
bereavement, 19
Beta brainwaves, 139
blood pressure, 81
blueberries, 112
boredom, 137
boundaries, 33
breathing signature, 89
broken heart, 81
cardiovascular, 91
caution, 17
Chakra meditation, 22
chant, 93
chanting, 109
child's pose, 87
Chloe Goodchild, 110
Colors
    aqua, 97
    green, 76
    indigo, 116
    orange, 43
    red, 30
    violet, 133
    yellow, 62
communication, 97
constipation, 33
cough, 81
crown chakra, 132
Dance, 56
dark energy, 98
decision making, 132
Delta brainwaves, 139
diabetes, 64
diaphragm, 89
digestion, 67
disappointment, 81
discernment, 137
DMT, 115
earache, 119
ego, 136
Einstein, 99
electromagnetic spectrum, 11, 133
Elements
    air, 77
    earth, 31
    ether, 98, 117, 134
    fire, 62
    water, 44
Émilie du Châtelet, 93
empathy, 80
endocrine system, 115
equanimity, 78
eternal youth, 161
feast, 55
fish, 57
fluoride, 119

fontanelle, 132
GPS, 115
gratitude, 93
green vegetables, 94
headaches, 119
heart, 75
heart chakra, 74
Hormones
    calming, 78
    endorphins, 84
    feel-good, 75
    female, 159
    serotonin, 128, 133, 139
    stress, 78
Humility, 165
IBS, 64
immune system, 139
Inner Guru, 115
insomnia, 136
integrity, 61, 101
journaling, 126
kidneys, 64
letter, 110
libido, 48
licorice, 112
listen, 111
love, 74
lucid dreaming, 115
lullaby, 109
lungs, 75
martyr, 33
meditation, 21
melatonin, 115
menopause, 49, 159
menstruation, 159
meridians, 12
metabolism, 97

migraines, 119
mirror, 163
miscarriage, 53
moon, 118
mudras, 18
overwhelmed, 48
parathyroid, 97
pelvic floor, 53
perineum, 53
pessimism, 119
pineal gland, 115, 119
pituitary gland, 115
post-partum, 159
posture, 158
prana, 63, 78
pregnancy, 49
presence, 61
psychotic, 119
puberty, 49, 115, 159
quantum physics, 133
quintessence, 98
Recipes
    earthy soup, 40
    easy chia dessert, 149
    Love Cookies, 94
    Sensual Salad, 58
    throat soothing tea, 112
    Visionary Salad, 129
    Yellow Sunshine pie, 71
reflexology, 61
Reiki, 18
religion, 132
Root chakra, 29
sacral chakra, 43
Sanskrit
    Ajna, 117
    Anahata, 79

manipura, 63
muladhara, 29, 32
Sahasrara, 134
Svadhishthana, 46
Vishuddha, 100
self-conscious, 109
self-esteem, 64
self-love, 89
self-pleasuring, 54
seven-chakra system, 14
sexuality, 53
Shakti, 118, 134
shame, 75
Shiva, 134
singing, 92, 109
sinuses, 119
solar plexus chakra, 61
solitude, 49
Sound healing, 18
Sounds
  AUM, 128
  HAM, 111
  LAM, 39
  OM, 147
  RAM, 70
  summary, 155
  VAM, 57
  YAM, 93
speaking your truth, 101
sphinx, 87
stiff neck, 19
stomach ulcers, 64
stress, 90
subtle anatomy, 14
survival, 29
sushumna, 13, 159
swim, 54

thenakedvoice.com, 110
Theta brainwaves, 139
Third Eye chakra, 115
throat chakra, 97
thyroid, 97, 101
tinnitus, 101
tonsillitis, 19
toothache, 101
tropical fruit, 57
truth buddies, 111
Truth telling, 110
turban, 132
unconditional love, 79
Unity, 166
universal love, 74
vagina, 53
vision board, 126
visions, 116
Vitamin D, 133
walk, 55
weight gain, 33
wheeze, 81
windsofdiscovery.com, 161
writer's block, 102
Yoga postures
  alternate nostril breathing, 124
  boat, 66
  Bridge, 52
  camel, 88
  cat-cow, 86
  chakra balance, 158
  chakra scan, 154
  chakra walk, 159
  child's pose, 67
  child's pose, 120
  Eagle, 123
  easy pose, 35, 83

Fire breath, 65
forward bend, 105
head tapping, 143
headstand, 141
heart opening, 85
Kali power flow, 50
Lion, 88
meditation, 138
mountain pose, 103
neck stretch, 106
ocean breath, 104

palming, 121
root lock, 38
seated forward fold, 122
sphinx, 87
throat opening, 104
thunderbolt, 37
twist, 67
ujjayi breath, 104
Up and down flowing dog, 51
warrior 2, 108
wheel, 88